Foundations of Noetic Medicine

Practicing the Medicine of the Mind

A monograph:

Foundations

of Noetic Medicine

Donivan Bessinger, MD, MS(Surg), FACS

Practicing the medicine

of the mind

Bessinger, (C.) Donivan (b. 1936)

Foundations of Noetic Medicine:
Practicing the medicine of the mind

Includes notes, references, bibliography

Library of Congress Control Number: 2009906565
ISBN 1-4392-4818-4

BookSurge Publishing
amazon.com

Foundations of Noetic Medicine

CONTENTS

Introduction (7)

Part I. A Medical Reality Check

Concepts (11)... Cosmos (20) ... The Quantum Cosmos (23)
Psyche (25) ... Dimensionality (28) ... The `Extra' Dimensions (29)
The Dimension of Thought (31) ... Consciousness and Nonlocality (33)

Part II. The Nature of Nonlocality

The Nuocontinuum (37) ... Comparing Nonlocal Theories (40)
Towards a Synthesis (46) ... P-time (50) ... P-time Dynamics (52)
Time for Eternity (54)

Part III. Healing Thought

The Philosophic Milieu (57) ... Reality / Physicality (59)
Causality / Probability (60) ... Complementarity / Superposition (62)
Homeostasis and Healing (65)... Healing and Complementarity (67)
Research Implications (68)

Part IV. Noetic Practice

Art of the Cosmos (73) ... Soul and Medical Art (74)
Psychoneuroimmunology (77) ... Placebo Power (79)
Health Yourself (81) ... Mindfulness (82)... Healing Intentions (84)
Medical Spirituality (90) ... Medical Intuition (93)

An Afterword (97)

Notes, References (101)
Bibliography (110)

Foundations of Noetic Medicine

Donivan Bessinger, MD

Introduction

Noetic medicine refers to the study and practice of the mental aspects of healing. The term appears only recently and rarely in the medical literature, but it has been a concern of healers throughout history, albeit within mainstream medicine well-hidden for a century or so. The discoveries by quantum physics in the twentieth century have deeply challenged notions of cosmos, but have hardly at all been assimilated into biology and medicine.

In particular, the discovery of a nonlocal realm, which lies within (and beyond, and under) the familiar relativistic spacetime physical realm, has forced a renewed inquiry into the place of mental techniques within modern medical practice. Perhaps more importantly, it fosters a search for a new paradigm or model within which certain unexpected "anomalous" results can be understood. Clearly, the several studies suggesting that prayer can favorably influence at a distance the probabilities of healthcare outcomes do not fit within the frame of the prevailing mechanistic biomolecular medical worldview.

The present study explores a most basic question: What kind of cosmos would it take to allow nonlocal results, not only at the quantum level, but also in the complex levels of the stressed human organism? The answer could have profound influence on our entire approach to healing, for it would address our most basic notions of individuality and of the relationships among all things at all levels. It would redefine our concepts about the connectedness of objects, and the notion of objectivity itself.

The term *noetic* is derived from the Greek noun, *Nous,* meaning mind. In current usage, the term refers to mind in both its conscious and unconscious, and individual and collective, aspects. Anaxagoras used the term to connote a Universal Mind as the basic reality, thus merging the ideas of mind and spirit into one.

The scope of noetic medicine is much broader than the study of clinical techniques, for it is a field which faces its own unification problem. For several decades now, physics has been occupied with a search for a theory of everything. In physical terms that translates to the search for a theory which unifies relativistic effects and quantum mechanics (quantum gravity). Since modern medicine is deeply grounded in the idea that physical reality is primary in healing, any change in foundational ideas about the physical world has immediate implication for theories of medical practice.

Further, since medicine deals with human *experience*, it confronts directly the problem which in the 1990s became the focus of a new interdisciplinary science of consciousness. Its so-called hard problem is nothing less than the problem of harmonizing theories of both physics and psyche. The prevailing view has been that consciousness is a mechanistic epiphenomenon, emerging from the physical organization of the brain at a certain level of complexity. However, the new physical knowledge exposes a profound paradox: (1) If consciousness is a physical phenomenon, it must have the quality and character of physical reality; (2) physical reality has been shown to be nonlocal; (3) therefore consciousness cannot be merely a mechanistic (local) epiphenomenon.

Physics has found that a unification theory is more intractable than first hoped, and the prospect of a unifying theory of physics and psyche must be even more so. Clearly, at this stage any such theory must be highly speculative. Many seem to think it inappropriate to try to span gaps in knowledge that are wider than a single foot-step, and do not trust apparently flimsy bridges of thin string to span chasms of the unknown. Yet it is the emerging clinical evidence which keeps driving the process, and evidence-based medicine must honor all evidence, however inconveniently removed from its current step-stone.

In this inquiry into nonlocal medicine, we will review briefly those ideas which are requiring a re-framing of our medical worldview, and then try speculatively to get it all together into an intuitive interim picture which is consistent with current evidence. The picture will be impressionistic, in which some areas are fuzzier than others, and necessarily will change with time. In a special sense, it may be more metaphorical than actual.

As we shall see, noetic medicine adds a new dimension to healing practice, while in no way diminishing concerns for physical evidence and appropriate physical interventions. However, even if the speculative synthesis to be presented proves ultimately to be wrong, the process can at least be helpful in defining the issues, and in shaping future inquiry. It will be well worth the effort even if it only helps practitioners become more sensitive to the noetic aspects of healing practice, and more conscious of interactions between the mental-spiritual worlds of patient and healer.

Part I

A Medical Reality-Check

Our concept of the physical cosmos has vastly changed in the years since Copernicus saw that the center of the universe was not the earth. Now we have telescopes which seem to be able to detect light almost as old as the universe. Since Descartes, as our science has reached farther toward the limits of the small and the large, we have thought of the universe as entirely materialistic and deterministic. We consider that our immensely large and complex cosmos has developed everything from planets to blossoms to brains, and that everything within it could be measured, if we could have just the right gauge.

It is somewhat ironic that as our concept of the physical cosmos has grown larger, our medical "cosmos", or concept of the whole of the human person, has contracted. To many people within medicine today, the *psyche* (the "soul" of Plato's day) is merely the product of the mechanistic molecular workings of the brain. Our *biomedical model* is a tightly framed picture with little room for such concepts as soul or spirit, and our concept of cognitive mind is computational.

Now new knowledge from a number of disciplines has left us with many concepts which do not fit within the prevailing medical model, nor into a mechanistic understanding of the universe. Our expanding "collective brain," the very science on which we based our *faith*, is fracturing that frame within which we have worked so comfortably and confidently. Somehow we must bring these new concepts into a "golden frame" by which we relate to the physical cosmos, and to the cosmos of the human person, including ourselves.

In our specialized professional world, most physicians have not had reason to be exposed to the technical aspects of quantum physics and the other sciences which will bear on our discussion here. Fortunately, it is not necessary to have a grasp of the technical details of those fields; we need only a few succinct concepts or lessons drawn from them. Let us begin by reviewing briefly and topically some of these helpful new concepts from physics, mathematics, depth psychology, and consciousness studies. Then we will able to link them into a new picture without needing exhaustive and unfamiliar technical detail, but only logic and intuition.

Nonlocality refers to a new understanding of physical reality. Here, *reality* refers to the most basic level of Being. The "local" reality is the world of ordinary phenomena, in which signals are limited by the speed of light, and force is mediated through a field and diminished over distance. Physicist John Bell showed (in Bell's Theorem) that if that were the only reality, certain experiments must show a mathematical inequality. Yet the experiments do not show that result. Experiments have now been done which show that correlated photons react together instantaneously even if miles apart. No speed-of-light signal could explain such a correlation.

Reality is **nonlocal**.[1] Physicist Nick Herbert writes

Bell's Theorem shows that the holistic grammar of the quantum formalism reflects the inseparable nature of reality itself. Beneath phenomena, the world is a seamless whole.[2]

Singularity — The mathematics which describes Einstein's theory of general relativity encounters situations in which the density of matter becomes infinite, thus breaking down at that point any mathematical description of the laws of physics. Such a situation is found at the center of a black hole.[3]

Hyperspace — The search for a theory which unifies the physical forces and the symmetries (e.g. the law of the conservation of energy) has led to a theory of seven or more dimensions in addition to those of space and time.[4] These dimensions need not be thought of as dimensions of "space" in which one might travel, but they represent degrees of freedom permitting actions within, and throughout, the cosmos. These extra dimensions must also be thought of as nonlocal since they are active at all points in space and time (e.g. the law of the conservation of energy is valid everywhere). Inconveniently, experimental confirmation of this theory would require a level of energy very close to that existing near the time of the Big Bang.

Probability — Quantum events are not determined by familiar mechanistic rules. Events must be calculated by probabilistic formulas. According to the current "standard model," an outcome may not be known until there is an act of observation. That is, only an interaction with consciousness, which collapses (or reduces) the wave function of the probabilities, establishes the reality of the quantum interaction.[5] Wojciech Zurek (Los Alamos National Laboratory) has shown that the environment surrounding a quantum system can itself "monitor" some of the system's observables, and thus be the *observer* which collapses the wave function.[6]

Complementarity refers to the particle/wave duality of "things" at the quantum level. The elemental thing may be seen as wavelike or particle-like: the *truth* of the situation does not rest with one or the other, but in the superposition of both states. Of course, choosing a method of observation involves an interaction of the physical reality with consciousness.[7]

Uncertainty always exists about a particle's momentum versus its position. One may not make a precise measurement of both at the same time; measuring one sacrifices the precision by which one may know the other (Heisenberg's uncertainty principle).[8]

Nonlinear dynamics, or chaos theory, demonstrates that there is order within systems previously thought to be random or unordered. Many functions exhibit *strange attractors* which act as though "an entity" were pulling a constantly varying output toward a coherent pattern.[9]

Fractal geometry is the geometry of fractional dimensions. Instead of the "design by chance" imagined by the mechanistic model, there seems to be an abstract mathematical reality underlying many familiar natural formations, such as the branching of bronchioles, ferns, plant stems, wave patterns, clouds, and shorelines. The Mandelbrot set, said to be the most complex structure known to mathematics, seems truly to be a geometry of the infinite.[10]

The limits of computability — In examining the question, simplified as *Does the set of all sets contain itself,* Kurt Gödel provided a mathematical proof that there is a limit to computability. The abstract ("mental") realm of mathematics, which is used to describe and model physical reality, has its own "nonlocal" limit.[11]

Microtubules are cytoskeletal structures of nucleated cells, especially well organized in neurons, and are apparently capable of responding to quantum-level events. Stuart Hameroff, MD, (Department of Anesthesiology, U. Arizona) and Roger Penrose, mathematician and physicist (Oxford University) propose that large blocks of microtubules produce consciousness by working in concert to "collapse the wave function" of quantum probabilities.[12]

Nonlocality in biology — Biology has strongly rejected the idea of a "vitalistic" principle operating beyond the reach of molecular mechanics. However, the genome of many species has been defined without revealing a basis for morphologic patterns. Botanist Rupert Sheldrake has postulated a nonlocal "morphogenetic resonance." His 1981 book was roundly dismissed in the journal *Nature* as "the best candidate for burning there has been for many years."[13] In 2001, *Nature* published a report of lines of evidence supporting nonlocality in biology. For example, though protein synthesis is governed by genetic mechanisms, protein folding is not. The shaping of proteins follows a relatively small set of abstract patterns (cf. fractal patterns, above).[14]

Anthropic principle — The mechanistic model of "design by chance" finds no room for theories of a purposeful universe. However, the laws of nature are so finely tuned that the slightest difference (e.g. in the gravitational constant) would have prevented conditions suitable for the emergence of consciousness. Thus, as Stephen Hawking notes,[15] it is exceedingly improbable that the emergence of consciousness is an accident. The fact that we are here to observe the cosmos suggests that there is a purposeful, or at least meaningful, link between cosmos and consciousness.[16]

Consciousness is a problem in several ways. Clearly it requires a functioning brain, but how does it arise within the brain? How is it that some patients can report specific and verified aspects of their resuscitation, even though at the time they were clinically dead? Or who, emerging to clinical consciousness after apparently having been "locked in" a vegetative state, report having been aware of events around them? What is the relationship between consciousness and the clinical unconscious of depth psychology? How could we explain the ability of a consciousness to describe itself? How is the unconscious content made conscious? Why does the existence of consciousness seem to be intimately related to the deep structure of the universe, as implied in the anthropic principle and in quantum theory? How could a mechanistic theory describe any of this?

Collective unconscious — Carl Jung's theory of a collective unconscious[17] has been almost universally rejected within academic circles. Yet, to deny a "phylogenetic" or collective aspect to the human unconscious is to deny an instinctual basis for psyche. It would require explaining why and how humans are exempt from a species-wide instinctual behavioral component which is present in all less complicated species. The question really is, to what extent is the collective aspect also nonlocal.

There is, of course, a "diffusionary" or cultural contribution to the content of myth, dream image, and hallucination, but prime questions remain. What is the ultimate source of the symbols which diffuse? Why is it that these symbols, even though culturally determined and diffused among cultures, are processed in highly consistent ways across cultures and across centuries, as Jung's scholarship and that of others has shown?[18] The proving of a nonlocal reality by physics requires taking a new look at the theory of a nonlocal psyche, especially if we are to think that psyche is determined by physical reality.

Archetypes — In Jung's theory, dream symbolism follows consistent patterns, defined as *archetypes*.[19] While there might be an instinctual (genetic) component involved (perhaps in "junk DNA"?), we might also imagine archetypes as nonlocal abstract entities, functionally like the strange attractors of nonlinear dynamics. These tend to hold a constantly varying output to a consistent pattern. In psyche, the functions will be expressed as images taken from personal experience in the culture. Archetypes, like mathematical functions in physics, need not have physical existence per se, to be integral to process ("output").

Precognition. Even though rare, clairvoyant or precognitive dreams and waking intuitions, (in which some level of information is "transmitted" across sometimes great distance between two people not otherwise in contact, but who are generally already known to each other) are elements of human experience which can only be explained by a nonlocal theory. The fact that such consciousness is rare does not dismiss the problem. The nature of cosmos must be such as to allow even the rare effects which occur, unless we are to postulate an "unordered cosmos." That of course is a contradiction in terms, for the Greek word *kosmos* means *order*.

Dream — The existence of the dream is itself problematic for the theory of an only-physical reality. How and why would the "selfish genes" of mechanistic evolutionary theory evolve the capacity for dreaming? If they do, why the great variation in level of dreaming among various people – some regularly dream quite vividly, some casually and sporadically, and many who do not dream at all (or perhaps, do not remember that they do). To what aspect of reality is the dream (and particularly, a precognitive dream) a survival adaptation? If it is such an adaptation, how is the "information" transmitted to the dream? Perhaps from the probabilistic information structure of quantum mechanics?

Synchronicity is a strikingly meaningful but ***non-causal*** connection between events in psyche and in the physical world. Occasionally two people who are emotionally close experience shared "synchronistic" moments even when separated by great distance. As in precognition, this too implies a nonlocal "communication" not unlike the nonlocal interaction between correlated photons separated by great distance. Neither situation can be accounted for by a mechanistic theory.[20]

Global consciousness, so called, spooky though it sounds, is a phenomenon newly recognized in science. Since 1998, a multidisciplinary collaboration of scientists, engineers, artists and others has been operating The Global Consciousness Project,[20a] collecting data from a network of random event generators, distributed globally. Data are transmitted via internet to a server in Princeton NJ, then archived. The data base is "interrogated" by investigators according to various hypotheses, asking basically whether certain events, widely known or not, correlated with a statistically significant variation from randomicity during the same time period. Strongly significant variations have been recorded during a number of events of intense interest, such as the two embassy bombings (1998), and especially on September 11, 2001. More benign events have also been correlated with the effect, such as a papal visit to Israel (2000), and US election events in 2008.

Is this a special large-scale example of synchronicity? The investigators offer no consensus theory in explanation of the effect.

Distant healing — A weak and variable effect of prayer on healthcare outcomes has been reported in several medical studies, [21] and perhaps may best be thought of as a special case of conscious intention and synchronicity. It is a *nonlocal* effect which cannot be accounted for by a spacetime signal. Of course, it can also be thought of as a theistic intervention. From the standpoint of theistic faith, the question is "how does God work", and it is as valid to analyze the effects of conscious intention as to analyze the effects of gravity. From the standpoint of non-theistic faith, the question is "how does Cosmos work". Whether, and to what extent, there is an effect, is still debated. The influence of study design and of investigator effects on outcome remains unanswered.

How then can we bring all of these anomalous effects into a consistent frame of reference? What is the nature of the reality in which such effects can occur?

Cosmos

If we are to remain true to science, we must integrate the data which science provides us, and be willing to follow where the process leads. All of the considerations just reviewed make it increasingly apparent that physics requires us to acknowledge *meta* considerations, that is, considerations which lie above and beyond the physics of matter and mass. Those of us biomedical practitioners who base our work on physics cannot disparage as "merely metaphysics" a *meta*-physics to which physics itself points.

Cosmos is the general descriptive term for all-that-is, which we have come to understand as an organic system of inter-related nested subsystems.[22] Its most ancient representation in art is a circle. In our ordinary positivist view of things conditioned by science, the term denotes only the material nature of the universe, governed by the laws of physics. In the ordinary local cause-effect world, time-distance relationships apply, and the speed limit is that of light.

However, as noted, the experiments validating Bell's Theorem[23] establish that "underneath" ordinary spacetime phenomena there lies a deep nonlocal reality in which none of these limitations applies. If we were to diagram cosmos as a metaphorical circle, we might add an inner concentric circle to represent nonlocality, but cosmos, as the term is currently used, would identify only the outer material "shell" of our experience of physical things. We have no agreed technical term for that which is "more" than matter, or beyond or outside it, or inside it.

Psyche has scientific validity as a psychological term. It denotes an inner personal dimension representing that aspect of experience which is normally unconscious to us, but which nevertheless influences individual human behavior. However, in ordinary usage, the term psyche (soul, spirit) has no meaning apart from the individual human personality. To speak of the soul or spirit of matter (one hardly dares do so publicly) does not compute. Yet, now physics says there is a nonlocal more to the matter-work of cosmos, and that domain is somehow related to the existence of consciousness.

There needs to be still another inner concentric circle, or at least a center-point. Cosmologists are beginning to speak more openly about a purposeful cosmos. For example, Hawking has asked, "Why does the universe go to all the bother of existing?"[24] If science is to ask "Why" as Hawking does, it must seek the "meaning" of matter. But *meaning* ordinarily has no significance in science. To speak of meaning is to speak of significance, connectedness, and order beyond superficial appearances. To speak of meaning in relation to the cosmos is to speak of metaphysics, the realm of religion and philosophy.

Yet, such meaning is implicit in the anthropic principle of physics,[25] in the strange attractors by which order emerges from chaotic chemical and nonlinear mathematical systems, and in the interaction between the quantum probability (wave) function and consciousness. Though such meaning is an idea new to modern science, religion and philosophy have variously described it as *logos, tao,* Way, and Word. Bergson called it the *élan vital.* It resides too in the "lure" orienting change mentioned by Whitehead, [26] and in the function of the radial energy of which Teilhard spoke. [27] Now, on scientific grounds alone, our "cosmogram" must have at least three compartments, if it is to encompass the phenomena of the universe. Resolving and explaining these relationships may be quite complex; or perhaps surprisingly simple, given a sufficiently large perspective.

The Quantum Cosmos

The search for a unified physical theory led to a continuing proliferation of proposed particles. In particle theory, a new messenger particle (or class of particles) called the Higgs boson [28] seems to be needed to explain how particles acquire mass, and to avoid the infinity terms (the result of a division by zero) which crop up in the formulas which unify the forces. Leon Lederman, experimental physicist and Nobelist, calls it "The God Particle." He wrote expansively, "The Higgs field, the standard model, and our picture of how God made the universe depend on finding the Higgs boson." [29]

Much more promising has been string theory, which posits the most fundamental thing as very small *strings* of diameters on the order of magnitude of the Planck length, 10^{-37} m. That is well beyond the reach of experimental confirmation, unless they are extended enough to be detected at the threshold of quantum effects, around the 10^{-17} m level. In order to account for the unification of the known physical forces, including gravity, string theory imagines a hyperspace of seven or more "extra" dimensions enfolded (or *compactified*) into ordinary space. However, there many variations of string theory. Harmonizing them requires a new field of study, called M-theory, which is still being investigated. [30]

Smolin,[31] whose research approach is *loop quantum gravity,* recently summarized loop theory, string (and M) theory, and quantum black hole thermodynamics (which points to a holographic principle). If the *loops* (at the Planck length, 10^{-37} meter) are taken to be the fundamental physical object, and thus constituents of *strings,* Smolin predicts that all of the three approaches can be harmonized into a final theory. That final theory would include a space structured in discrete Planck-scale units, which is nonlocal and relational, and which is best understood in terms of process rather than mechanistic, objective states. He predicts that quantum theory eventually will be reformulated into a theory of information. Thus, major questions remain. Oxford mathematician Roger Penrose has written,

> *If there is to be a final theory, it could only be a scheme of a very different nature. Rather than being a physical theory in the ordinary sense, it would have to be a mathematical principle whose implementation might itself involve nonmechanical subtlety.* [32]

One of the principle problems in quantum physics is the question of observer effect. What is the role of consciousness in resolving the uncertainties of actions at the quantum level? Before an observation, the question of whether a quantum event has occurred can be resolved only by calculating a probability. The unconscious reality of the event is that it is a mix of the probabilities that it has happened and that it has not. That wave function of probabilities is said to collapse only at the point of observation, that is, only in the interaction of unconsciousness with consciousness.

Schrödinger [33] illustrated the problem by describing a thought experiment involving a cat sealed in a special box: If the quantum event happened, the cat would be poisoned; if not, when the box was opened, the cat would be found alive. Until then, we could know the result only as a calculation of probabilities. Under the conditions Schrödinger described, we may think of the cat's condition only mathematically: the cat is both dead and alive, with equal probability. Only by the interaction of event with observer is the "wave function collapsed." (The process is also referred to as *reduction* of the probability wave function, and *decoherence* from the superposed state.)

If a tree falls in the forest when there is no one present to hear it, has there been a sound? That question can be resolved by adjusting the definition of sound. In the question of the quantum "event in the box" we are dealing with something much more fundamental. Can creation occur without an observer? Without consciousness? Or at the least, without an infinite principle connecting all-that-is? That may be the most basic question which begs resolving.

Psyche

Psychology is conventionally defined as the study of behavior, but for our purposes, it must be returned to the meaning implied in the roots of the word: the study of soul and spirit. Of course, the most obvious phenomenon of psychology is the emergence of consciousness. In the light of the anthropic principle of physics, we now must ask, as a distinctively psychological question, what purpose for the cosmos does consciousness serve?

Another question: Jung[34] has presented the evidence for an archetypal collective unconscious which, from a mechanistic standpoint, would have to be inherited as the base-content of human nature. Archetypal genetics has yet to be defined. Symbol processing certainly does have its "local" physical aspect, in the function of the brain and the whole-body physiology which supports it. Nonetheless, that there is a nonlocal reality undergirding psyche is readily evident.

The reality of the dream experience is nonlocal, unconfined by rules of time and space and normal effect. Further, it is nonlocal in that the reality extends beyond the individual, consistently following patterns evident throughout the recorded history of dream and myth. The psyche functions as though the brain, or at least its apparatus of consciousness, is "observer" for the dream "event in the box" of an unconscious nonlocal collective reality. The archetypal unconscious suggests that there is a psychological substrate from which consciousness and its content have emerged.

In the emergence of consciousness primally, and in the extension of consciousness in modern people through the dreaming process, the collective unconscious (self) seems to serve a nonlocal integrating function, yielding images which the conscious (ego) must differentiate from its "local" observations of the external spacetime world. Thus is consciousness extended.

In that process, however, the ego must self-reflectively also *keep in mind* that our perception of the external physical world is not the reality of the physical world, but an interpretation of it; nor is the external phenomenal world the only reality. To keep our interpretations of the physical world "honest," we must subject observation to tests of consistency and reason, but the calculus of consciousness is the calculus of whole process, both differential and integral. Consciousness cannot be extended, but is diminished, when it denies the reality of the unconscious.

Jung has also pointed to certain meaningful associations between events in psyche and events in the physical world, but which are not related causally. He called such an association a synchronicitiy, which he defines as "an acausal connecting principle."[35] These simultaneous or closely associated occurrences are not connected physically, in any ordinary cause-effect way. However, they are connected meaningfully, that is, psychically. They may have very powerful impact on a person's psychic state and on the subsequent unfolding of personality. Jung studied them with Wolfgang Pauli, a quantum physicist in whose life such phenomena were frequent.[36]

A synchronicity seems to suggest that a nonlocal psychological reality either communicates with or is identical to the nonlocal reality known in physics. Since it is inconceivable to have two *nonlocal* realities coexisting separately from one another, we can confidently assert that there is indeed, only one nonlocal reality.

Another set of phenomena inviting consideration is that which includes group hysteria and mob action.

A classic example is that of a high school band on a bus trip, on which all members get "food poisoning" simultaneously before a big game. After exhaustive epidemiological work, no evidence of infection or toxins is found, and the "cause" is attributed to stress and the power of suggestion. The mechanisms are entirely unconscious to the band members; it is as though their psyches have "communicated" in a way that makes them act together. Similarly, in mob action, though the members may be conscious of the anger which moves them, generally the event seems to be loaded with an unconscious dynamic within the group which prepares the way for and perhaps amplifies the event itself. (Such a nonlocal mechanism would help explain the intractability of such major problems as the Middle Eastern conflict and global terrorism.)

Dimensionality

Physicist Paul Davies has written that one of the basic problems is constructing an adequate definition of dimensionality.[37] The ordinary dictionary definition describes a dimension in terms of magnitude or direction (height, depth, width), and we ordinarily think of the dimensions as perpendicular to each other. But that works only for the familiar spatial dimensions and the actions of ordinary objects. Imagine compressing all of three-dimensional space toward a single point; as it comes close to a point, the concept of being perpendicular loses all meaning. Another problem is that it does not really make sense to think of time (which is a dimension, too) as perpendicular to anything.

A dimension is one of the domains of action permitted to or on an object. By domain I mean something like a field of influence or action. For example, verticality is not a force which acts on an object, but is rather an abstract permissive feature which in some sense "shapes" a configuration or movement in space, and which influences our description of the movement. But the abstract is real! Take verticality away from three-dimensional space, and an object is permitted to move only in a way that we can analyze as a mix of lateral and forward-backward motions. Take the lateral away, and the object may move only along a straight line (one-dimensional space).

The `Extra' Dimensions

The "string" theories,[38] which approach a "Grand Unification" of all of the physical forces, posit dimensions beyond the four of spacetime. There is no theoretical limit to the number of dimensions, for external to spacetime there is no concept of "container" or limit.[39]

Since all of the nonspacetime dimensions, by definition, are not extended in space or time, we must conceive of them as represented by points. Since they act together on spacetime, they must "intersect" or somehow communicate with the primal spacetime point. For that reason (and because in the absence of spacetime no point can be offset from another), we must imagine the dimensions as many points superimposed into one. Let's call it the superpoint. Such is the nature of a *singularity*, the point at which the laws of physics and dimensions break down. We may imagine as many superimposed points (dimensions) as past and future experiments might require to explain the phenomena of cosmos.

The initial conditions of our spacetime universe are defined in that one superpoint/singularity. The Big Bang represents the explosive expansion of four of those dimensions, spacetime. The creation-energy (superforce) responsible for that expansion is concentrated in and at the multi-dimensional superpoint. Yet we must also think of other changes at the superpoint, for as energy levels dissipate immediately after the Initial Event, the superforce quickly "evolves" into the four physical forces conventionally known.

We have said that only the spacetime dimensions are expanding, because the force dimensions ("contained" in the superpoint) are not spatial. By definition, we may not imagine non-spacetime points as extended in space. However, all points in expanding spacetime must still "communicate" with the force dimensions (and the symmetry dimensions, but we are neglecting them for the moment). All points in spacetime must intersect the force dimensions.

It is as if the force dimensions too have been expanded to the size of spacetime, for they can act on any particle of energy/matter in the universe. One might imagine that one point has been stretched as a featureless elastic sheet, a continuum in which the dimensional point is everywhere the same.

However, quantum theory deals with these forces as discrete waves/particles acting in spacetime. For example, the force of gravity is communicated by gravitons; the strong nuclear force by gluons; the electomagnetic force by photons. If we conceive the stretched points of the dimensions as "sheets," the sheets must have waves in them. It is these "stretched sheets" which constitute the field in which energy interacts with particles to sustain (and indeed, to continue the creation of) the universe. As I once expressed it in a poem, it is the field "where the forces play pinball / with gravitons and gluons / and modulate / the all."

The Dimension of Thought

Let us imagine again that spacetime (four dimensions) is compressed toward a point. It is futile to ask what is outside that small pellet of spacetime, for the concept of "outsideness" has no meaning except in respect to some frame of reference within spacetime. As the pellet becomes smaller still, it shrinks toward nothingness, for a point is an abstract concept of zero dimensions, not extended in space or time, and thus it cannot "contain" anything. At that point, nothing exists except the thinker who is trying to imagine nothingness.

If we could model thought as only an epiphenomenon of matter, reached at a certain degree of complexity, it has no fundamental reality of its own. In that case, our thought experiment to shrink the cosmos reaches a point at which thought is extinguished, and the experiment must stop, if it is to follow the rules that it is modeling. However, by accepting that thought might have a reality of its own, and by considering the problem from a whole-system perspective, we were able to continue the thought experiment to the point at which only the thought remains. The epiphenomenon idea is not an adequate model of reality, since we can indeed continue the experiment under the conditions outlined.

This "negative proof" is indirect, serving only to eliminate the epiphenomenon model. It does not prove that there is an independent and fundamental reality beyond spacetime and matter; the experiments investigating Bell's Theorem do that. This line of thinking, however, does lead us to suggest that thought is a primary aspect of reality. It seems that cosmos itself is saying with Descartes, "I think, therefore I am." Or as his statement has been interpreted, "I am conscious, therefore I am." [40]

Because of this inescapable "relativistic" connection between cosmos and thought, I cannot imagine creation *ex nihilo* (from nothing), for the concept of nothing always collides with the existence of the one who is the thinker. *Nothing* has no meaning apart from something. The dimension of thinking is required to imagine zero-dimensional spacetime.

The epiphenomenon model posits that *nothing* (literally, "no *thing*") is defined as the absence of matter. If that is so, thought is nothing; but if it were *effectively* nothing, I could not be thinking that thought, so thought must be a something. Thus, we must say also that thought has reality, for it has effects. After all, saying that effects can occur from that which is un-real would be meaningless—a special kind of singularity, perhaps, in which all meaning breaks down! There can be no nothingness, for even if all which exists is reduced to no-thing-ness, a dimension of reality remains. Reality requires at least one dimension in addition to spacetime and that reality seems inseparable from the dimension of thought. Thus are we led to a rather extravagant and intuitive proposal, following Anaxagoras: Thought is the missing particle, the missing dimension.

Consciousness and Nonlocality

Quantum physics already acknowledges the importance of consciousness as "observer." Consciousness is the substrate of thought. Thought is consciousness dimensionally extended, whether in time or some other dimension. Thought is process. Any unification of the laws of physics must necessarily take into account the thought/consciousness dimension, and thus must unify physics with psyche as well.

In his book *The Self-Aware Universe*, Amit Goswami[41] uses the term consciousness to mean a transcendent consciousness, which forms (or is) the nonlocal reality. Other physicists seem to define the term less carefully, and one often wonders whether a given text about observer effect is referring to ordinary individual awareness, or to some more general property of reality.

As a clinician, I would prefer another term, for it is useful to preserve the important distinctions between consciousness as it is experienced by the patient (i.e., *subjectively*), as it is experienced by the practitioner (*subjectively*), and as its effects are observed clinically (*objectively*). There is also the important distinction between consciousness and unconsciousness.

Psychologically, ordinary human consciousness is the subjective realm of ego and the cognitive functions called mind; and neurologically it refers to a patient's observed state of awareness. The clinical unconscious is the realm of psyche, with both personal and collective aspects. Perhaps better language will come along in time. Until then, let me suggest interim language for envisioning relationships between matter and psyche.

Suppose that there were a unit [42] of psyche; to continue the language of particle physics, we might (whimsically) designate it the *nuon*, from the Greek word *nous*, for mind. The "nuon" would represent the dimension of thought which exists in (at, as) the superpoint defining the conditions at the Initial Event. As in the domain of the force dimensions, the nuon must be imagined to expand as a field or continuum as the spacetime continuum expands, a "stretched sheet" with "waves" which is also nuonic (or *noetic*). Let us call that realm the *nuocontinuum*. The nuon of the superpoint is extended in spacetime in a way conceptually (abstractly) analogous to the action of the forces.

Yet the extended nuon must also be construed as the domain of the symmetries, such as the principle of conservation of energy, which are nonlocal. That is, they are everywhere in effect, without being constrained by the speed-limit of light. The nuocontinuum thus represents a multidimensional bridge between forces, symmetries, and spacetime. The nuocontinuum is the *collective nuon* containing all potentialities, but the collective is the unit, itself the symmetry which unifies the forces and symmetries. The nuon is the "infinity particle" which "solves the formulas."

Thus, the nuocontinuum may be thought of as the realm of fractals (fractional dimensions) such as those which give the mathematical order to the "chaos" images, or as a Hilbert Space, an abstract mathematical structure (an infinitely dimensioned array), which is the realm of probablities of the Schrödinger equation.[42a]

Or, perhaps one might prefer to think of it as the prime tone of which the symmetries and the forces are harmonics. Whether construed mathematically or poetically, the abstract nuocontinuum is the "space" containing all the information necessary to create a universe, but a universe which is organically creating itself.

Human awareness, which occurs at a level of extraordinary complexity in the organization of spacetime particles, would involve, not a *creation* of consciousness as an epiphenomenon, but a sensing of a quality which is already there, as the reality-dimension of the cosmos. The observer effect at the quantum level (and the health of Schrödinger's cat) is then to be understood as an interaction, not with a particle of concrete matter, but with the reality substrate from which matter arises.

If we construe the whole nuocontinuum (rather than the experimenter) to be the "observer" of the quantum event in the box, we avoid much of the confusion and exasperation which Schrödinger's thought experiment evokes. Hawking wrote, "When I hear of Schrödinger's cat I reach for my gun!" [43] Even Einstein was repelled by quantum uncertainty. DeBroglie especially held out for an interpretation of quantum physics which supported concreteness. We rebel against the idea of a universe based on uncertainty, and we seek to assure ourselves that what we experience is a concrete reality.

However, if the nuocontinuum is the observer which resolves the quantum uncertainty, our own individual sense of uncertainty is also resolved. The collapse of the particle wave function (the coming into being of the particle at a particular point in spacetime, i.e. the "stablization" of a transient *virtual particle*) would be a function of the nuocontinuum acting as a whole and over several instants of time, rather than as a local observer. The nuocontinuum is the observer who actualizes creation—the cosmic event in the box—thus answering the problem of "whose consciousness", prior to the development of individual consciousness. It is that cosmic observer who unifies the quantum effects of the electronuclear forces and the cosmic effects of gravity.

Part II

The Nature of Nonlocal Reality

The Nuocontinuum

We have suggested that nonlocal reality can be represented as a *nuocontinuum* which is "mindlike" in several senses: (1) it exists beyond the realm of matter and mass; (2) it is unrestrained in its scope of operation by time-distance relationships; (3) it is an infinite connecting principle which encompasses all that is; (4) it is the realm of the effective "observer" who on the whole-cosmos level resolves quantum probabilities into actualities; and (5) it is the reality base from which individual consciousness emerges.

During the further discussion of these ideas, it will be helpful to keep in mind the vast scale of the cosmos, in terms of orders of magnitude (powers of ten):

10^{29} m, cosmos (~14.5 billion light years)
10^{6} m, earth radius (6,378 km)
1 m,   human height (~1.8 m)

   - - - -

10^{-6} m, erythrocyte (7 microns)
10^{-9} m, nanometer technology
10^{-15} m, proton
10^{-17} m, quark

   - - - -

10^{-37} m, Planck length

There is more room on the scale of magnitude lying below human size than beyond it. In the vast unknown of the domain between quark size and the Planck length, there is more room for organizational detail than between the quark and human scales, or about as much as between the scale of an erythrocyte and that of the observable cosmos. The "subquantum" Planck-to-quark scale is still within the spacetime realm. It is at Planck scale that relativistic effects must cease; beyond it lies nonlocality. Because of the relativistic time-dilation effects seen as motion approaches the speed of light, and from the Heisenberg uncertainty principle, we might expect that as subquantum scale approaches Planck scale, effects become progressively less *local*.

The nuocontinuum idea is necessarily a fuzzy one, and may include effects in the near-Planck region of the subquantum scale. Zeno's paradox reminds us that for any value an infinitude of halvings is required as we attempt to approach zero. Richard Feynman said, "There's plenty of room at the bottom." He was speaking of the possibilities of nanometer scale technology, but his statement holds true "all the way down." [1]

According to the complementarity principle, a quantum-scale object may be defined as either particle or wave, depending on the method of observation. Thinking about the nature of the subquantum realm is easier if particles are thought of as waves, or "energy knots."

There are complex interference patterns when sets of waves interact, resulting in still further wave patterns. These interactions also occur among the harmonic frequencies above and below the prime tones. We would expect there to be a very complex interference pattern which expresses the relationship ("correlation") between any two quantum objects. Any such "subtle" patterns among increasingly short harmonic wavelengths would become progressively more diffuse and indefinable in spacetime. They would tend toward nonlocality even though they expressed relationships among objects and complex clusters of objects within spacetime.

The Aspect experiments,[2] done in confirmation of Bell's Theorem, showed simultaneous changes of state in pairs of correlated photons, too far removed from each other to be influenced by a local signal. In the nuocontinuum theory, that would be accounted for not by the "physical" characteristics of the photon (or other quantum object), but by its nonlocal component.

The nuocontinuum is construed as an infinitely broad connecting principle, which integrates all physical and psychic states of the cosmos across time. As a particular organization of quantum objects traces its "lifeline" of physical existence, it will also make a "trail" of correlations which will intensify its "image" within the nonlocal reality. Yet, the nuocontinuum also contains within itself the potentialities for all physical and psychic states. All pasts and all futures nonlocally exist together, enfolded in a holonomic way (i.e., like a hologram). The particular future which is brought to pass through operations of the physical world will organically cohere with the state of the whole.

Comparing Nonlocal Theories

The idea of a nuocontinuum broadly overlaps, and very near-ly superimposes, with several important theories of nonlocal reality offered for discussion. However, expressing nonlocal-ity as nuocontinuum has the potential to shed further light on those theories, and to bring them further toward unification.

Bohm: quantum ontology

The idea that the nuocontinuum is a "hologram" in which each object is a relational expression of the whole is consis-tent with Bohm's description of a holonomically enfolded (im-plicate) order.[3] Further, it complements the Bohm and Hiley *ontologic* interpretation of quantum theory.[4] In contrast to the "standard" *epistemological* model (in which the state of a system is "real" only when the wave function is collapsed by measurement or other conscious observation), they hold that the particle has an objective being, that it is an actual-ity whose probabilistic behavior derives from a "pilot wave" which guides it in one or another channel of possibilities, and accounts for interference patterns observed in double-slit experiments.

Bohm and Hiley also consider that an elementary particle "has a complex and subtle inner structure." Such subtle structure might easily be accomodated within the scale be-tween the particle's size and the Planck length, which is of about the same order of magnitude as that between our own size and the particle's.[5]

The Bohm and Hiley equations demonstrate nonlocal influences which would be consistent with the description of the nuocontinuum. Since the quantum potential contains the same term in both numerator and demoninator, "it does not necessarily fall off with distance." In one-body systems, the particle's behavior "can depend strongly on distant features of the environment." In a multi-body system, "the behavior of each particle may depend nonlocally on the configuration of all the others, no matter how far away they may be."[6]

Zurek: Decoherence and environment

Wojciech Zurek of the Los Alamos National Laboratory further developed the idea that the environment surrounding a quantum system can "monitor" some of the system's observables. In that view, the environment itself can act as the observer which collapses (decoheres) the wave function.[7]

The nuocontinuum idea is consistent with his work, in that it would be the connecting principle by which the environment registers its observation. Each interaction would then be "computed" to its place within the whole. This would be a quantum interpretation which, like Bohm's, is *realistic*, harmonizing local and nonlocal aspects of physical reality. Zurek has provided a glimpse into "structure" within the sub-Planck (*nuocontinuum*) region. Non-linear quantum systems have nonlocal effects there, and these features influence the sensitivity of the system to decoherence.[8]

Goswami: science within consciousness

The idea of a nuocontinuum is entirely consistent with physicist Amit Goswami's model [9] of nonlocal reality as a transcendent/immanent unitary consciousness, but there is more to account for than mere awareness. Nonlocal reality has a dynamic, expressed in the result of its "computing" through the processes of local physical reality. (Note that in this computer metaphor, it is not the nonlocal reality, but the physical spacetime actuality which is the "hardware" whose state is changed and in which information is stored.)

For example, consider that a synchronicity [10] often involves some sudden, dramatic, and otherwise unexplained physical phenomenon. The relationship is noncausal in ordinary spacetime terms, but even so the appearance is that something "mental" (i.e. nonphysical) "made it happen." Nonlocal reality seems to have some quality of "mind" or meaning beyond mere awareness.

This distinction having been made, the nuocontinuum and the unitary consciousness models can be superimposed. Goswami's terms "idealistic science" and "science within consciousness" would be equivalent to speaking of science practiced within awareness of the nuocontinuum.

Sheldrake: habits of nature; morphic fields

Biologist Rupert Sheldrake has advanced a theory of the formation of organisms (and inorganic forms) under the influence of morphogenetic (or morphic) fields. Though he does not explicitly name a fundamental nonlocal reality, nevertheless he writes, "Morphic resonance involves a kind of action at a distance in both space and time. The hypothesis assumes that this influence does not decline with distance in space or in time." [11] Thus the reality implicit in the theory is that of *field,* which he defines as "non-material regions of influence." [12]

Further, "Morphogenetic fields are 'probability structures'...". And, the process "is analogous to composite photography..." [13] In a personal communication with the author (September 1996), Sheldrake writes that he thinks in terms of local morphic fields connected by nonlocal morphic resonance.

The effects he describes could be clarified by the concept of the nuocontinuum. If there were a holonomic nuocontinuum connecting every quantum object (and all the nested formations of them), it would not be necessary to postulate multiple "fields." The physical reality of cosmos is itself the storage medium of multiple forms, and all the rest of developing cosmos always has access to it through the nonlocal holonomic "coupling" of the nuocontinuum itself.

The representation in the nuocontinuum of that *form* stored in cosmic experience would be an idealized blend of all similar forms, as indeed occurs in composite photography. When multiple observers rate blended faces for beauty, the score gets progressively higher when more faces are included in the blend.[14] Through the nuocontinuum, morphogenesis has access to the "most beautiful" composite expression of experience, but under local influences the form will not be copied exactly. However, with each new physical variation, the composite of cosmic experience with that form is slightly altered, so that further evolution of that organism is "pulled" in a slightly different direction by the holonomic composite. That is, it tends toward a holonomically idealized version of itself. Organisms in relatively stable niches experience less alteration from the composite over time, so would have less "pull" toward change. In that view, "Darwinism" itself seems to involve a blend of both nonlocal and local influences.

Sheldrake also argues in favor of laws of nature as having the nature of habits, rather than being immutable preexisting characteristics of the universe. In the nuocontinuum concept, all current experience is coupled ("unified") with all previous experience. The physical laws can be understood to be the influence of that unified experience bringing any object and combination of objects into consistent patterns of behavior. And that, of course, is an acceptable definition of habit.

Hameroff and Penrose: human consciousness

The new science of consciousness has become a very active field of inquiry, but the field is very far from any hint of consensus. One of its most interesting new theories would require the concept of something like the nuocontinuum, and it describes a possible link between the local and nonlocal aspects of mental experience.

The proposal deals with microtubules, which are cytoskeletal structures present in nucleated cells but especially well organized in neurons. Anesthesiologist Stuart Hameroff and mathematician/physicist Roger Penrose [15] propose that microtubules are the physical site which interfaces with a nonlocal reality to produce consciousness, through a process they name *orchestrated objective reduction*. Within the microtubules, subunit proteins called tubulins can register quantum-superposed states, remain coherent, and recruit additional units "until a mass-time-energy threshold (related to quantum gravity) is reached." [16] The quantum probability wave function is thus collapsed ("reduced") . They side with those who view reduction as a "real" physical process (rather than a purely abstract or metaphorical one). Hence, *reduction* is *objective,* and awareness arises through time-dependent concerted (*orchestrated*) action of blocks of microtubules.

The physical neuro-psychic apparatus is thus coupled with a level of reality which they describe as consistent with the idea of panpsychism; with Goswami's theory of the primacy of consciousness ("monistic idealism"); and with the descriptions of consciousness as "occasions of experience" (Whitehead) and "moments of experience" in meditation (Buddhist texts). Further, it is a realm of "non-computable" effects.

They write, "Our viewpoint is to regard experiential phenomena as also inseparable from the physical universe, and in fact to be deeply connected with the very laws which govern the physical universe." [17]

Towards a Synthesis

Though we have now established a perspective from which to attempt a synthesis of physics and psyche, various questions remain. As Penrose noted, [18] any satisfactory theory of consciousness must ultimately connect up with a theory of reality. Yet that consensus theory of reality is still elusive. Various physicists have suggested that the sought-for theory is likely to be simple but decidedly unconventional. In Part I we mentioned Lee Smolin's recent predictions about the shape of a final theory. Earlier, Smolin [19] suggested that the unification likely will also require a new understanding of time, and must account for extraordinary organic complexity, in addition to its unification of quantum theory and relativity.

A truly *final* theory must also unify physics with psyche, since both domains relate to nonlocal reality. [20] All of the major physical theories so far focus on the most fundamental discrete features of space, but the complexity of their mathematics puts such solutions out of the reach of an ordinary intuitive understanding of cosmos. Thus, any final theory will require some sort of metaphorical interpretation, if it is to become a working theory in healthcare practice.

There seems to be a philosophical way around his dilemma. The considerations mentioned do not clarify the nature of time, though Julian Barbour has argued in favor of "instants of time", rather than an "arrow of time", as the fundamental time-reality.[20a] By focusing on the tiniest features of time, rather than of space, we may be able to create an intuitive theory which works for visualizing the relationships between physics and psyche in healthcare practice. Such a result would serve us well even in the absence of a final physical theory. To achieve that, we must step boldly across the broadest part of the conceptual chasm. Even so, let us attempt a trial solution which would relate the problems of dimensionality, time, nonlocality ("eternity"), quantum probability, and gravity. Clarifying these relationships, even metaphorically, should help better define the reality-context in which consciousness studies and our healing actions must take place.

Our first step is to accept the findings of quantum physics as normal features of the universe. These findings are "weird" only with respect to mechanistic theory, and only to the extent that their implications have not yet been accepted.[21] The next step then involves focusing on certain questions about the nature of (1) nonlocal reality; (2) the speed limit of light; (3) dimensionality; and (4) time/duration.

(1) Nonlocal reality: "Local" reality is the familiar spacetime world of classical physics, with its speed limit for signals and diminution of force over distance. Though phenomena are local, quantum physics says that reality is *nonlocal*, as established in experiments affirming Bell's Theorem. Further, according to the dominant interpretation, the law of conservation of energy applies everywhere in the universe. From that, we may infer that the nonlocal domain must provide (or be) a steady-state reserve of energy available for the creation of mass ($E = mc^2$), and for translation into local actions of all types. But what is the relationship between local and nonlocal domains?

(2) The cosmic speed limit: Presumably an illuminated cosmos without a speed limit would be perceived as a blinding glare, and time would be a meaningless concept. There could be no distinction between local phenomena and nonlocal reality. We take the speed of light as a given, as a defining parameter of this cosmos. But by what "mechanism" does cosmos, based in nonlocal reality, establish a speed limit? What is the limiting factor?

(3) Dimensionality: The definition of physical dimension seems to be slippery. One theory suggests they may disappear at highest energies.[22] We ordinarily think that there are three discrete dimensions of space, and time yet another dimension, all operating as a continuum. In this discussion, *dimension* is simply a permission to move or to have an effect, *i.e.* a degree of freedom; but the "licensing scheme" confers cumulative privileges: With a two-dimensional license one may be stationary (zero-D), move along a line (1-D), and on a plane (2-D). With three-dimensional privileges one may move anywhere, spatially speaking (3-D), but requiring time to do so; thus, local reality is four-dimensional. Also, string theory and its variations treat forces and symmetries as dimensional, thus requiring that cosmos be a "hyperspace"[23] of at least eleven dimensions.

Yet our degrees of freedom are also constrained by prior events. We may not move in ways or make combinations of things for which the history of cosmos has not prepared a potential. For example, at the macro level, it is premature for me to book a flight to Mars, but each increment in space technology helps prepare the way for someone to do so, someday. Each increment in the organic complexity of cosmos increases its degrees of freedom, and like dimensionality ordinarily construed, does so cumulatively and exponentially. Should we not then consider whether the evolution of dimensionality itself is a basic feature of cosmic evolution?

(4) Time and duration: Time measurement in the local domain is relativistic; we might refer to that as Einsteinian time, or "E-time." But, according to one's state of consciousness, perception of time passing does not necessarily correspond to E-time—it is strikingly variable. Whitehead[24] referred to reality in terms of discrete "actual occasions" or "actual entities," each of which "experiences" how its world is qualified by other actual entities. The extension of these *occasions* of *experience* would represent a psychological time (all *experience* being psychological, even when unconscious). Let us designate that as "W-time," which some cultures (predominantly Eastern) have construed as cyclic, and others (predominantly Western), as linear.[25]

Time's arrow for both E-time and W-time is reversible. But time's arrow for cosmos points one way, so some new conception of time (or new relativization of time) must be forthcoming. Bergson theorized that duration (*durée,* connoting especially continuity) is the key feature of "creative evolution", which carries its own forward impetus, or *élan vital*. Whitehead dealt with time/duration as the "extensive continuum" of the actual entities, both authors emphasizing that being is process of becoming. Is it possible to conceptualize a one-way cosmic time which is consistent both with relativistic E-time and with quantum duality and uncertainty? [26]

Kabir, giving voice to the Eternal, wrote, "You will find me in the tiniest house of time." [27] That is the direction toward which we now look for a synthesis.

P-time

Imagine a "protocosmos" consisting of nonlocal Energy, which somehow contrives to express, by the simplest possible rules, its potential for the type of physicality we know in our own experience. Such a physical cosmos could be "programmed" to operate by these three rules. For that universe as a whole:

(P.1) The life of the cosmos is a series of discrete states;

(P.2) Each new state determines the probabilities which govern the next state; and

(P.3) Each new state confers a new degree of freedom (dimension).[27a]

Hilbert space is an infinitely-dimensioned mathematical structure.[28] Running the above program by discrete increments (P.1) creates a growing (abstract, conceptual) Hilbert space, but one in which each new dimensional state enfolds its predecessor (P.2), yielding an "implicate order" (*cf.* Bohm [29] and Bohm and Hiley.[30]) That would mean that the momentum and all other historical characteristics of any quantum object would be represented in the multi-dimensionality of the current state of cosmos. The smallest interval imaginable in current physical theory is the Planck time, a natural unit defined by the speed of light, but it is unimaginably infinitesimal: 10^{-43} seconds. Let us construe the extension of the discrete dimensional states into a series (P.1) as the "ticking" of the "Planck clock."

Such a ticking could represent a synchronization pulse between nonlocality and locality, but cosmos offers no external reference against which such a mechanism could yield a timing. Even though the "P-clock" is not really a clock, the pulsing of nonlocality would represent the critical interaction between the nuocontinuum (the realm of the quantum world's *potentia*) and the physical actuality realized through quantum-level process.

Each Planck time "tick" (P.1) (one can hardly avoid calling it a "plick") would re-seed the probability wave function (the Schrödinger equation) to determine the distribution of the whole-cosmos Energy for each momentary (re)creation of mass (P-3). A "sum over histories"[31] would be inherent in that process.

There would also be a speed limit for physical objects (photons), since nothing may move faster than the P-clock, each plick being 10^{-43} sec (Planck time). Timing (E-time) can become apparent only as motion is tracked within spacetime, from plick to plick. A speed limit of light is inherent in that process. The Planck interval would be the fundamental parameter, from which all other physical parameters derive.

In such a pulsed-nonlocality cosmos, physicality (locality) exists only during each plick. The interval between the plicks, being nonlocal, would be undefinable and imperceptible.

The state expressed (P.2) at each dimensional increment would include the characteristics of all interference waves at all harmonics among all clusters of quantum objects. Since the probability wave function of local-level interactions would be renormalized to nonlocality (zero point field) at each plick, cosmos would in effect be the observer who reduces its own wave function. This is consistent with Zurek's work on quantum decoherence by the environment.[32]

P-time dynamics

The probability would become extremely high that an atom would continue in existence as an element of the same type, or if it were an unstable element, would decay in a probabilistic way. For an object consisting of many atoms/molecules, the probabilities that it would tend to retain its present state of motion would be so high as to give rise to a "law" of inertia.

For a complex system, especially a life system, the P-clock rules would result in a growing (large scale) probability of expressing some new degree of freedom (P.3) as a new characteristic. We could think of that as an "impetus" (*élan*) which could be expressible as a probabilistic state vector. The inherent probabilities also favor its returning (smaller scale) toward its stable historical condition (P.2) after perturbation. There would always be tension between emergence and equilibrium (physiological homeostasis), as we observe.

Something similar would be seen at the cosmological level, in the tension between expansion and gravity. From our "local" perspective, the relationship between gravity and spacetime is now construed as topological: Space is a physical matrix deformed (curved) by mass, yielding gravity effects.[33]   That fosters a search for a contrary expansive force preventing cosmic collapse.

The pulsed-nonlocality idea offers the possibility of a probabilistic view in which expansion of the universe is analogous to *emergence*, and gravity analogous to *homeostasis* as described above. In the momentary renormalization and (re)creation of all states of matter (with cumulatively higher probabilities), new degrees of freedom (P.3) could increasingly and most easily be expressed as further elaboration of whatever (of quantum scale, 10^{-17} meter, or subquantum scale) is found to constitute the matrix of space, [34] resulting in further separation of galaxies.

Gravity is the observed effect of accelerated motion (Einstein's equivalence principle), as seen within spacetime. In the pulsed-nonlocality model, a particle in motion (or a large cluster of particles) is recreated across a "quantum gap" at each plick. The probabilities (P.2) governing its new position have a component derived from its historical momentum, but also a component representing the resultant of the interference wave patterns of all harmonics (including any which may exist at subquantum wavelengths) between any two mass objects. (These are presumed from the wave aspect of the wave/particle duality.) The intensity of such interference patterns would be proportional to mass. These characteristics will also be conserved by the process (P.2), as though the two objects were attracted.

If we presume also that the state actualized at the next plick represents the best fit of probabilities computed non-locally across the cosmos (the "world equation"), the observer in spacetime will see motion (relative to his own state of motion), not as uniform, but as deflected as though by a force which was in tension with the vector of expansion. The gravity vector would predominate in dense regions of space, while the expansion-vector would dominate in low-density regions. (But we must note Penrose's reminder[35] that the nonlocal state vectors express, not simple probabilities, but complex numbers.)

Time for Eternity

Such a schema, taken as a theory of the current cosmos, would be rather startling. Cosmos would be "neorealist" in the sense that it is "really there" even in the absence of a human or other sentient observer to collapse the (probability) wave function. But human consciousness, expressing its own degrees of freedom in various ways, would be one aspect of the state of cosmos being integrated at each plick. It would thus be interactive with cosmos with a potential to affect nonlocally, in subtle but unconventional ways, the probabilities governing local states.

It has been proposed that consciousness is achieved by quantum-level interactions within the brain, through the neuronal microtubules,[36] or through boson condensates in brain water.[37] The new view offers the possibility of understanding consciousness as a diffuse sensing by quantum mind of cosmic integration within nonlocality, providing a screen on which local content is projected by processes generated at ordinary neurological scale. In any case, the P-time idea would have a number of interesting implications for consciousness studies, as well as medical practice and other fields.

When ideas leap too far ahead of current evidence, the standard response is "naked speculation." This proposal, being philosophical more than physical, is more in the line of a naked intuition, which would be even harder to prove than quantum gravity. After all, it will be difficult to describe it mathematically, for mathematics abhors infinities. (Quantum theory even discards them, through the process of renormalization.) Nor would it be easy to derive testable predictions from it. It seems that the idea must stand or fall entirely on the results of testing by thought experiment.

Though such an idea may be valuable only as metaphor, it is intriguing that it provides an intuitive resolution of the two-slit paradox (in which an interference pattern appears on a film plate, as though there were two beams of light, even if only single photons are projected): Given stable conditions (this experimental situation) in which two paths remain equally probable, the succession of plicks would actualize pulses of energy randomly in each of them, resulting in the observed interference pattern.

The pulsed-nonlocality idea highlights critical reality issues in the search for an understanding of consciousness, including medical experience. One might also hope that discussing such ideas will help science-based medical practice reestablish a relationship with its ground of being, however we name it or construe it in our many cultural traditions. Doing so requires extending our frame of reference beyond the local domain. The pulsed-nonlocality idea offers a new view of the richness of the ground of being in the nonlocal mix of energy and *potentia* [38] in the nuocontinuum, interactive with the physical and psychic states of being in each moment. There's a great deal of poetry in such a concept, but poetry itself is another level of consciousness. [39]

Part III

Healing Thought

The Philosophic Milieu

It is probably fair to say that the discussion so far seems to have little connection to anything we think of as "medical." So, what's the point?

Actually, that *is* the point!

We have reached a point at which our prevailing medical thinking is disconnected from what is known about nonlocality in the physical world. For a profession which bases itself on evidence of physical reality, such a disconnect is a disruption, a wound in its body of knowledge which calls for healing if the profession is itself to be healthy. It seems natural to refer to that process of re-examining our relationship to reality as *healing thought,* in which we heal our thinking so as to think more comprehensively about healing.

Just as the cells of the body flourish (or become stressed) in a fluid *milieu interieur,* so does our healing practice live in a philosophic milieu, which appropriately relates a physician to the patient, to the practice environment, to the base of knowledge, and to the physician's own sense of self. Such a world-view is multi-level and inter-disciplinary, and is based on various interactions and adaptations of physicians to life systems. Thus does medicine maintain an equilibrium between its technologic skills and its humanistic concerns. [1]

Ever since the 1980s the medical profession has seen itself to be in some sort of "crisis" [2] Usually we analyze our situation in terms of issues related to managed care, medical liability, or governmental and other third-party regulation. However, it often seems that a significant portion of the energy invested in those discussions arises out of the often-expressed sense of dis-ease about the philosophic milieu of practice, and a sense of loss of meaning and connectedness with our patients and among ourselves. Our way of thinking is integral to healing those issues. A new way of thinking, harmonizing all knowledge and experience, could vastly expand the possibilities for the future of healing, and would doubtless improve our satisfaction with our calling.

The new way of thinking will involve recognition of new inter-level relationships, which within science have heretofore gone un-named. The idea of nonlocal reality is an important example. The "eternal" (non-spacetime) realm has been named variously in our many different religious traditions, but use of any one of those terms within science carries connotations which the scientific method cannot evaluate, much less affirm. Thus *nuocontinuum* is offered as a non-weighted generic secular term, which specifically connotes nonlocal relationships to physical (and psychological) action. Though the term could be interpreted within theology as denoting the realm of providential or karmic action, its use as a scientific (medical) term is not meant to convey a theological meaning. Let us examine how some of the questions raised by the new physics relate to the philosophic milieu of healing practice.

Reality / Physicality

From the mechanistic point of view, *reality* equates with the physical world of discrete historical space-time events. The *mental* world is accommodated by the epiphenomenon idea which we have previously discussed. The mental world is the world of image and imagination, fantasy, and perhaps *virtual reality,* which can be taken to mean either un-real or *as if* real. We subscribe to this sharp divide between the physically "real" and the mentally "un-real" despite the fact that all *experience* is mental. Our experience of the physical world is not of the physical world itself, but of an interpretation of it, processed from various kinds of afferent neurological information. That entraps us in a perceptual paradox.

The public too, our patients, have bought into this mechanistic equation of reality with physicality. A broader, more wholistic view seems to be growing more rapidly among patients than among healthcare professionals. Even so, many patients still commonly expect and insist upon an obvious physical intervention even when the physician recognizes that the symptom is a stress-mediated somatization from some situational problem. Such a diagnosis is taken to mean that the problem is "all in the head" and thus unreal. It may be taken as a rebuff, with a feeling that the physician has not taken the patient's problem seriously. More significantly, however, that reaction can block a patient's self-examination of the relationships between lifestyle and health. Equating reality with physicality, whether by patient or physician, leaves no conceptual room for any healing other than a pill or procedure. The concept of the *nuocontinuum* acknowledges the reality of both physical and mental-spiritual aspects of experience, so that all influences which bear on healing, direct and indirect, can be considered.

Causality / Probability

In the mechanistic view, all causation is linear, as though any effect is mediated through discrete links in a chain of action. That one-dimensional view is made two-dimensional by consideration of branching cascades of activator actions, as in Krebs' cycle, the coagulation cascade, or carcinogenesis models. [3]

The life-systems view of Bertalanffy,[4] which is applied to medical practice in Engle's *biopsychosocial* model,[5] adds the third dimension, by considering the complexities of feedback loops among all levels of organization. Nonetheless, it too is a mechanistic view, in which all action, regardless of complexity, is construed as causal.

These same considerations operate at the clinical level, in the search for direct linear connections both in diagnosis and treatment. Because of variability of outcomes, we evaluate results of treatments by probabilistic methods. However, we do so under an unspoken assumption that a direct deterministic answer should have been possible, were it not obscured by the complexity of the situation, which harbors "hidden variables." We have not taken variability of outcomes as reason to doubt our basic doctrine of causality.

Quantum mechanics, however, forces an entirely different view. At the most basic level of the currently known forms of matter, all physical events occur probabilistically. The Schrödinger equation by which quantum events are predicted analyzes the complex *vectors* which contribute to the action. However, as in the example of his famous cat, the outcome is not known until a measurement is made, that is, until there is an act of observation. Further, nonlocality implies that events cannot be isolated so as to have an only-local significance. If it is the "environment" which determine the action, that environment must include properties of a *nuocontinuum*. In other words, the environment is cosmos acting nonlocally as a whole. If all actions can be analyzed as based on physical reality, then actions at all levels are subject to non-locally resolved probabilities, with at least some degree of uncertainty of outcome.

Probabilistic uncertainty is a basic feature of cosmos, and is not consistent with a mechanistic/deterministic worldview. That understanding fosters a change of attitude and a more humble approach to healing. The physician who realizes that "interventions" do not directly control outcomes, but only influence them probabilistically, is better positioned to evaluate all factors bearing on a clinical situation. The physician's bearing and attitude influence the probability of a good outcome, as do the patient's own mental-spiritual attitudes toward the illness and many often-hidden life issues. Those variables factor into the outcome strongly or weakly, and may enhance or diminish the desired effect of the physician's intervention.

The mechanistic mind-set often seems to resort to a basic over-simplification: We expect the chain of causation to yield the most-probable outcome, and we are surprised when confronted with the improbable. In clinical work, we typically analyze problems in terms of simple probabilities. If we were to view clinical situations as though they were quantum events, from both a probabilistic and nonlocal perspective, we might become able to refine the precision of evaluation of study outcomes and prognosis. That would involve encoding information about the magnitude and direction of many relevant factors into complex vectors such as are used in the Schrödinger equation. Even so, uncertainty of outcome is inherent in the system, and a result can never absolutely be known in advance of an event.

Complementarity / Superposition

Quantum theory confronts us with the notion of duality: The quantum object exhibits characteristics of both particle and wave, but both features cannot be observed at the same time. It seems to be one or the other, depending on the method of observation, but what is seen is not a complete description of the object. Both characteristics must be taken together as the best representation of the truth of that particular state. Similarly, there is complementarity in the representations of quantum probabilities. In the Schrödinger cat example, before an observation (measurement), the only available representation of the truth of the situation is that dead and alive are superposed into one complementarity, resolved only by an observation.

Nadeau and Kafatos[6] have pointed to a number of other complementarities encountered in physics and mathematics, such as time/space, matter/energy, field/object, part/whole, zero/infinity, and real/imaginary numbers, which led physicist Niels Bohr to speak of complementarity as the "logic of nature." The apparent micro/macro discrepancy in modes of observation between quantum events and the larger-scale events of classical physics is itself a major complementarity which has made it difficult to see that the universe as a whole is a quantum object.

The complementarity principle bears noting in clinical practice, for no single clinical observation or diagnosis can provide a complete description of a patient's state of being. From the nonlocal perspective of the nuocontinuum, in the complexity of the human organism a vast number of states at all levels of description are superposed and integrated into levels of function which often compensate to remarkable degrees for various debilitating conditions.

The principle can also be seen to be operating in psychology. Jung[7] showed that humans fall into certain types or personality patterns, based on opposing pairs of characteristics. The general attitude (orientation) of ego-consciousness tends to be either *introverted* toward the unconscious self or *extraverted* toward the outer world. Incoming information is processed non-rationally by *sensing*, in an item-by-item fashion, or by *intuition* which works toward integrating source-data. Received information is processed by rational process, either by linear *thinking* or by non-linear valuing (or "*feeling*"). Humans have the capacity for all of the functions, but one or the other in each of these pairs is naturally preferred.[8]

In Jungian theory, archetypes are also viewed as paired opposites (feminine/masculine, mother/father, young/old, light/shadow, etc.). The lifetime process of personality integration (*individuation*) is to bring about a "coincidence of opposites" of the types and archetypes within ego-consciousness. This concept is enriched by understanding the "opposites" as complementarities which are always superposed, but actualized and expressed to varying degrees through life-process.

Healing thought is itself a complementarity which refers both to linear and non-linear processing of received information, about healing specifically and about the universe of knowledge. *Healing thought* is a participation in the nonlocal "logic of nature," by which all complementarities are resolved into the actuality of the cosmos as a whole. Nonlocality is equivalent to relationality, and is the whole-cosmos connecting principle. *Healing thought* is the essence of nonlocality, and the fundamental action of *nuocontinuum*.

Homeostasis and Healing

The dominant characteristic of life systems is flux equilibrium, which, at the level of the individual organism was named by Cannon as *homeostasis.* [9] For the organism, or for a whole system of organisms, survival requires the capacity to maintain a dynamic stability, on which depends the ability to heal wounds and to adapt to environmental stresses. Homeostasis is that well-tuned condition of least strain, in which the system as a whole survives and seeks to actualize its potential for development as a whole. We may use the term homeostasis to apply both to the flux equilibrium and to the processes by which it is achieved.

In life-systems theory, each subsystem is a whole contained within a boundary, but a boundary which is permeable (e.g. a cell membrane) affording input/output for communication with the larger whole of which it is a part. Wilber [10] has described that unit of the whole as a *holon*, which itself contains other holons. The holon is not merely an isolated part, but is an integrated equilibrating system which is a complementarity, being both part and whole.

From the nonlocal perspective, homeostasis is a probabilistic dynamic of holons, a *nuoflux* [11] in which the whole is held together by nonlocality itself. In the pulsed nonlocality model presented in Part II, the flux equilibrium lies in the sequence of probabilistic choices throughout the system, subject to all influences from within and beyond the (sub)system. However, if we look carefully, homeostasis is not merely a "holding sameness" as a flux equilibrium in the present moment. Any living system is drawn not only toward healing, but toward further growth and development. In some sense, homeostasis is vectored toward a goal specific for a level of the living system, and for the whole.

Because homeostasis is not mechanistic, its dynamic is non-linear, subject to unpredicted changes in the balance point, or *attractor* of the system. As has been mentioned, abstract principles govern protein folding, and fractal geometry is evident throughout biology in various unfolding patterns. Nonlinearity is beginning to be recognized in medicine, e.g. in gastric activity and the pathogenesis of arrhythmias,[12] and has been proposed as being a basic process in dreaming and consciousness.[13] The mechanism of irreversibility of shock, which acts clinically as though there had been a sudden shift of the *attractor* of the system, may well be related to non-linear inter-system processes.

In such a system of nested interactive holons, no one level can be taken as primary in its influence, a point which often seems to be lost in presenting the promised benefits of genetic therapy. Even DNA, which is itself subject to feedback loops and to injury and healing process, cannot be held out as a first cause of disease, but is only one level of action in a living system whose complexities ultimately are orchestrated in the nonlocal quantum system. In that sense, all healing is an effect of cosmos as a whole, and subject to many levels of influence and intervention, strong and weak, direct and indirect, conventional and unconventional.

Healing and Complementarity

The feedback loops which are characteristic of homeostasis are active within and among all levels of organization, not merely at the molecular level. From the perspective of the quantum-whole, homeostasis is the process by which the superposed complementarities of a system are nonlocally measured or observed while compensations are actualized to achieve a new coherence of the system.

The challenge of the healer is to assist that process by becoming conscious of ("measuring") the physical and/or mental light/shadow complementarities of the patient's situation, and to hold them non-judgmentally in superposition while intervening in ways which compensate toward a new coherence of the whole. The healer intervenes in various ways in the patient's system, but in doing so, the healer becomes part of that homeostatic system.

Intervening in a compensating way is the hallmark of the allopathic system of medicine. The allopathic approach provides a counter-balancing adjustment (of whatever appropriate type) which is vectored in a direction opposite to the effect of the disease process. However, in analyzing (diagnosing) the negative vector that is the dysfunction (the disease system), the healer mentally identifies the disease, and mentally *identifies with* it and the patient in a "homeopathic" way.

To the allopathic mind, the treating of physical disease by a diluted trace of substance which is "like" the disease makes no sense at all. Yet psychotherapists have referred to the "homeopathy of the psyche," meaning that the psyche's compensating dream images tend to be *like* (not opposite to) the distressing problem. It seems appropriate to say that the allopathic-homeopathic approaches are themselves a physical-mental complementarity, both of which are operative in the healer's work. It is this "homeopathy of the psyche" which may explain the otherwise inexplicable reports of salutary effect of homeopathic intervention.[14] This idea will be helpful in considering the placebo effect, in Part IV.

Research Implications

Practice and research in the biomedical model are based on the presumption that systems are localizable, that is, separable into discrete *objects* which are analyzable as distinct from the practitioner or researcher. The recognition of nonlocality completely undermines that presumption, and forces a change in the understanding of the relationship between subject and object. We commonly refer to persons being tested as subjects, but conceptually treat them as objects. Yet the nuocontinuum concept helps to understand that these "objects" of research really are subjects, who experience the test and experimenter subjectively.

A landmark study by Wiseman and Schlitz[15] has demonstrated that the researcher is also *subject*, who brings a subjectivity to the study which can determine the outcome nonlocally. In prior separate studies, each of them had studied whether "receivers" could detect the gaze (attention) directed at them by unseen "senders"; Schlitz had measured an effect, whereas Wiseman had not. They then collaborated in a joint study, in which each carried out the identical study design at the same facility using a pool of volunteer participants drawn from the same university population. Participants were studied in an unplanned, opportunistic sequence. Participants were stared at (or not) using video equipment, by the experimenter located six rooms away on the same floor of a psychological research laboratory. Electrodermal activity of the subjects, monitored continuously during *stare* and *non-stare* trials, was recorded by a password-protected computer system.

The study groups did not show a statistically-significant difference in questionnaire scores of *belief-in-psi* (extra-sensory perception), though the group tested by Schlitz had more subjects in the *belief* category.

The two experimenters had very different outcomes. The group tested by Wiseman, the skeptic, did not show an effect. The group tested by Schlitz, the proponent, measured a statistically significant difference in electrodermal activity between the *stare* and *non-stare* responses.

It follows that studies which show weak effects and variability of outcome must be evaluated for the possibility of nonlocal researcher-effect. Such may well be the explanation for the negative response in a widely publicized therapeutic touch study,[16] done by avowedly skeptic investigators. Similarly, unrecognized nonlocal effects might skew results in studies done by researchers who are enthusiastic advocates of their hypothesis, even when commercial incentives are not involved. Presumably this is a weak effect, of no direct concern in studies which reach high statistical significance.

The researcher-effect especially casts doubt on the validity of meta-analysis when it is used to validate a weak nonlocal effect, such as that shown in intentionality studies to date. Astin *et al.* [17] attempted a meta-analysis of five prayer studies, but found too much variability of design to proceed. Roberts *et al.* [18] did proceed with a meta-analysis of four prayer studies for the Cochrane Database of Systematic Reviews, with inconclusive results. Targ [19] has reviewed a number of considerations bearing on the design of distant healing research. It seems reasonable that the "fatigue effect," when a placebo or other treatment initially seems to work but then loses its efficacy, might be due (at least in part) to an intentionality influence by patient or physician.

The result of the Wiseman and Schlitz study also opens the possibility that nonlocal effect could potentially confound the blinding of certain prospective studies. The trait of clairvoyance seems rare in the general population at the present time, but a reliable estimate of prevalence is problematic, since many such people keep the trait private to avoid social repercussions. Inclusion of several unrecognized "intuitives" in a small participant group theoretically could confound an otherwise sound study design, and possibly skew its results.

Evaluation of unconventional therapies uncovers a number of other problems as well. As noted, the standard approaches to biomedical research are based on a presumption of objectivity, which nonlocality calls into question. We typically admit into practice those procedures which meet one of three types of evidence: (1) at least one properly randomized controlled trial, (2) non-randomized controlled trials, if results are repeatable in more than one center and consistent across time, and (3) the experience-based consensus opinion of respected authorities.[20] These principles are valid for all types of studies, but it should be noted that in Category 3, there has been the additional presumption that the findings must fit the established model of knowledge, otherwise the "authority" would not be "respected."

Thus there is a complementarity of sorts between experience and worldview, in which getting to the "truth" of a situation involves consideration of both. It bears repeating that noetic practice as discussed here is intended to be based on carefully weighed evidence, giving due consideration to safety, efficacy, and ethics. It is *alternative* only if the mainstream fails to bring the best possible integration of physical and experiential knowledge into its worldview and its practice. That *healing thought* brings us to Part IV.

Part IV

Noetic Practice

The Art of the Cosmos

According to current understandings of quantum physics, the complex design being painted by cosmic art is that of a creation-in-progress in which spacetime phenomena are actualized within and unified by a seamless nonlocal realm, which is inextricably correlated with consciousness. That worldview, derived from current evidence (and which stands regardless of the author's idea of *nuocontinuum* and speculation about pulsed-nonlocality), pulls the medical profession toward an entirely new interpretation of healing and practice.

The twentieth-century practice model (still well ensconced) focuses on repairing ("fixing") the biological mechanism at the most reductive level appropriate to the diagnosis at hand. For example, the current interest in gene therapy moves the focus of disease to the sub-molecular level. In this model, the healer is the fixer, the patient is passive observer, and there is no place at all for the concept of nonlocal or "spiritual" effect.

The art of the cosmos has drawn a profoundly different view. Now we must see the physician, surgeon or other therapist not as "fixer" but as helper, who uses specific *local* (physical) techniques as appropriate. It is the patient who is the healer, who cooperates as consciously as possible in restoring whole-organism homeostasis. The new model accepts that nonlocal, noetic means have an useful role.

It is particularly interesting that it parallels the traditional shamanic model, at least in that respect. However, there is a curious divergence, too: Though physician and shaman share a long apprenticeship in the physical ways of their respective systems, the physician is moved into a fragmented reductive world which tends to objectivize away the soul aspects of the patient-physician relationship, and of the physician's own self. It is not surprising that physicians, and particularly surgeons, are at very high risk for eventual dysfunction and impairment.[1] The medical system offers nothing comparable to the shaman's retreat into the wilderness, in the quest of a personal vision by which to integrate healing knowledge with personal meaning and purpose. For the physician, too, that somehow must become a personal quest, whether it leads to the wilderness or not.

Soul and Medical Art

Within science-based medicine, the word soul now "does not compute". If we think of it at all, we consider it a religious or spiritual concept which is best described mythopoetically. Dr. Albert Schweitzer wrote,

No one can give a definition of the soul. But we know what it feels like. The soul is the sense of something higher than ourselves, something that stirs in us thoughts, hopes, and aspirations which go out to the world of goodness, truth

*and beauty. The soul is a burning desire to breathe in this
world of light and never to lose it—to remain children of
light.* [2]

Psychotherapist Thomas Moore wrote, "It is impossible to
define precisely what the soul is ... We know intuitively that
soul has to do with genuineness and depth." He continues,
"The great malady of the twentieth century, implicated in all
of our troubles and affecting us individually and socially, is
'loss of soul.'" [3] In that sentiment, he echoes the theme implicit in the title of Carl G. Jung's 1933 book, *Modern Man in
Search of a Soul.* [4]

We might well say that *soul* is that great unknown of the unconscious psyche which can progressively be made known, at
least as a present and active dimension of mental life. After
all, *psyche* is the ancient Greek word translated by our word
soul, but *soul* has now lost out to *psyche* itself as our preferred
technical term. However, experience so far shows no hint of a
boundary to soul or psyche, however defined. Both words do
indeed involve us in "something higher", deep, and genuine
which daily seeks to give purpose and meaning to our work,
and which inspires us to communicate the same sense to patients in our healing practice. If connection to such soul has
been lost in society generally, it would not be surprising that
it should come to be lost in medicine as well. If both are true,
we could expect that healing the healing profession would, in
the process, make a substantial contribution to healing our
sorely stressed society.

Soul-based practice is often referred to as *holistic*. Yet, in today's intellectual climate, there are problems about calling such a worldview holistic. Many in the world of alternative medicine describe themselves as holistic, but place themselves in opposition to medicine's reductive approach. However, a true philosophy of the Whole is a complementarity which cannot exclude reductive research, for it is research into detail which provides the data by which we compose our concepts of the whole. A whole cannot exclude its parts. Any alternative which rejects or devalues the scientific and cognitive processes by which physical knowledge is gained and affirmed is not holistic at all.

It must also be said that the medical profession, if it is to regain its soul, must not reject or devalue the intuitive "spiritual" element in composing its worldview. That human nature is based on soul is amply evident in the fullness of its expression in art and religion throughout all cultures and throughout all history. A psychology which deals only with the cognitive, behavioral, or molecular aspects of human functioning is a superficial psychology, devoid of the essence of being human.

Reason itself requires that medicine embrace the fullness of the human person and potential, and that it deal at depth with *soul*. If we do less, we fail to meet the imperatives of reason and of whole-system homeostatic process. That is, we fail at healing. A healing approach which keeps both science and soul in homeostatic balance is fully holistic. A system which attempts to heal without soul is as out-of-balance as a system which attempts to heal without science.

Psychoneuroimmunology

Doctoring the soul is the literal meaning of the word psychiatry, but psychiatry's dominant view of itself now is as a "medical" rather than a "talking" specialty. Michels and Marzuk[5] write of the "profound transformation" in psychiatry's "major shift of paradigm." In psychiatry, "The focus of research has shifted from the mind to the brain ...". In essence, the pharmacologic treatment of mental illness (now conceptualized as *behavioral issues*) has become so successful that psychiatry no longer needs to focus on psyche.

During the same period there has been a substantial increase in the search for the physiological mechanisms for the "mind-body connection." The earlier *psychosomatic medicine* was mainly limited to the search for empirical correlations between physical diseases and psychological diagnoses. Expanded knowledge of cellular and immune dynamics, however, with further refinement of molecular research techniques, has fostered development of the new (or, newly named) field of *psychoneuroimmunology* (PNI), with an intensification of emphasis on physical mechanism.

The **P** of *PNI* is characterized largely by studies of stress, coping strategies, and cognitive and emotional states as they relate to physical manifestations of disease.[6] Stress has many effects beyond the long-known fight or flight responses, and is a significant factor in many disease processes. Stress effects include increase in skin permeability,[7] decrease in CD3+ and CD4+ T lymphocytes and interleukin-1 production,[8] decrease in natural killer cell levels,[9] and delay in surgical wound healing.[10] However, immunological responses vary according to perceptions of stress, ways of coping,[11] and levels of anger and cynicism.[12] Depression[13] and thought-suppression[14] are also associated with immune dysfunction.

Psycho-oncology is an active, but young, area of interest within PNI research. Spiegel *et al.* have shown a favorable effect of psychosocial support for patients with metastatic breast cancer.[15] In an overview lecture, pioneer researcher Steven Greer[16] reported that stress, hopelessness, affective states of mind, and personality "hardiness" all have tentatively been correlated with cancer effects. He summarized, "The biomedical model of disease, though powerful, does not explain all known facts about cancer," and he called for a new conceptual framework.

The broader concept of the P in PNI must be able to explain somatization,[17] by which the unconscious expresses itself in bodily symptoms, and explain the occurrence of spontaneous remissions[18] sometimes observed in patients who within the biomedical model are considered incurable. It must also explain nonlocal effects, such as the ability to influence electrodermal activity in a remote subject,[19] and prayer effects discussed below. A true integration of the elements of PNI awaits a breakthrough in understandings of nonlocal effect within consciousness studies. If physics itself has a limit to its mechanistic powers of description, so too must psychoneuroimmunology.

Placebo Power

Most of us recognize a potential placebo effect of medication. However, as the emphasis of medical practice has shifted to technology-based specialization, we have come to discount the "placebo effect" of a physician's personality. In a 1992 newspaper interview,[20] medical historian and author Edward Shorter of the University of Toronto spoke of medicine's general loss of skill in "evoking the placebo response" in interactions with patients. He indicates that the physician is often unaware of having such an effect. He attributes the effect to a high regard by the patient for the physician, and to the amount of time the physician spends listening to the patient; the loss of these qualities in medical practice has been accompanied by "the loss of medicine's therapeutic power".

The doctor-patient relationship cannot be examined or explained at the molecular level. The transference responses by which patient and physician relate is a complicated high-level effect, mostly unconscious, with both intra- and inter-personal dimensions. If something is wrong in medicine's collective interactions with patients, it must be a "soul-level" problem, involving our philosophic worldview, our attitudes about life and healing, and the unconscious dynamics of our own psyches.

Dr. Eric J. Cassell [21] (whose thoughtful humanistic approach is a valuable reminder of the ideals of doctoring in the era before managed care) wrote in 1976 of "the healing connection" expressed in a "silent language" of "tenderness phenomena."

Writing in an era in which Freud was much more influential, Cassell said that transference is a specialized usage of a normal bonding phenomenon, necessary to the individual for completeness or wholeness. He explained that we could just as well speak of connectedness, as long as we remain aware that the connectedness involves the whole range of the points of contact between two people, from thought to feeling.

The idea of nonlocality would not have been readily available to Dr Cassell in the mid-1970s, but nonlocality certainly validates the importance he gives to connectedness in the cultivation of the doctor-patient, helper-healing relationship. Cultivating the "silent" aspects of the healing connection is the essence of noetic practice. In the language of nonlocality, healing intentions, humility, empathy, and mindfulness together create a nonlocal *correlation* within the unconscious "psychic commons" between patient and physician, analogous to the correlation in which photons act together irrespective of the distance between them.

Noetic practice is also mindful of the healing environment. The ambience of the physician's practice setting is in some sense an extension of the physician's own presence, with potential to calm or further stress patients, who usually are tense and anxious about the medical encounter even before arrival. Too often in these days of computerized telephone answering, "music on hold" (and worse yet, commercial announcements on hold, or "health information" raising worries the patient had not thought of yet), jarring background music, high hospital and office noise levels, garish color schemes, bad art, and cold rooms create "industrialized" atmospheres which foster stress and alienation, rather than the confidence and serenity characteristic of healing relationships. Providing a supportive ambience may or may not by itself make a measurable difference in health outcome, but at least it can make it easier for the physician to project the placebo power of mindful practice.

"Health Yourself"

The idea of "healing with soul" confronts the physician with another type of reality check. Waldfogel has written,

Of course, to engage patients effectively in the spiritual realm, and thereby to offer better and richer support to ill persons and their families, the health care provider must possess a personal and spiritual maturity. [22]

In its essence that is a personal quest, and the richness of world culture offers many paths. However, there is much more that could be done within the medical profession to provide practitioners with appropriate non-sectarian peer support and to encourage personal spiritual development. We must find a number of ways to foster among ourselves the rediscovery of personal meaning in healing practice.

There is already a variety of national and regional conferences on spirituality and medicine, sponsored by medical schools and other health-interest organizations. One local effort known to the author especially seems to be a promising model which could be implemented widely. In 2002, the Dean

Medical Center[23] of Madison, Wisconsin, a multispecialty group of some 400 physicians, offered a series of physician-oriented events called *Health Yourself*. The program was set up as an evening "fair" with a variety of stations which member physicians might visit in sequence, to explore and discuss adjunctive methods which might benefit themselves and their patients. However as the name suggests, the emphasis is on helping themselves as individual healers to manage stress and come to terms with the deeper personal dimensions of medical/surgical practice. As organizers of such conferences almost universally attest, the response was enthusiastic.

There seems to be a considerable hunger among physicians for recognition and expression of the *soul* dimensions of healing. As the *Health Yourself* concept illustrates, measures which benefit patients may also benefit physicians themselves. Understandably, physicians usually prefer to pursue personal development in venues separate from their patients. Hopefully, the concepts offered in the following sections will help physicians organize personal quests and implement local group programs for the benefit both of physicians and their patients.

Mindfulness

In simplest terms, mindfulness is living in the experience of one's own mind. It is an ability cultivated by meditation, a practice known in various forms and taught in many cultures, ancient and modern, with spiritual, mental and physiological benefits.[24] Hayward succinctly described the method of meditation:

In practicing the method ... I sit with my legs crossed, my palms resting on my thighs, back straight, eyes open with gaze down. The practice is just to pay attention to whatever thoughts, feelings and bodily sensations arise to awareness, as they arise, and let them go when they want to go. The effort is to be direct and clear, not rejecting thoughts, feelings or sensations that feel bad (immoral, stupid, etc.), not trying to hold onto positive feelings or thoughts, nor to think any particular thoughts or follow a special train of thought. Being gentle with my thoughts and feelings, I try to be open to them, but not to encourage them unnecessarily, just to let them be there as they are. [25]

Hayward is writing from the perspective of Tibetan Buddhism, but with only minor variation, the method is the same in most established religious traditions.[26] Some emphasize the recitation of a sacred or personal word (mantra), while others do not. Benson[27] studied practitioners of transcendental meditation, in developing his method of "relaxation response." Findings included an antihypertensive effect, decreased oxygen consumption, and enhancement of the alpha-wave EEG pattern which is associated with relaxation but is different from sleep tracings. The mindfulness-based stress reduction and chronic pain clinic established at the University of Massachusetts Medical Center by Jon Kabat-Zinn[28] is based on the Vipassana ("insight") method from Theravadan Buddhism.

Epstein has provided a well-researched review of the benefits of mindfulness in medical practice. He summarized:

Mindful practitioners attend in a non-judgmental way to their own physical and mental processes during ordinary, everyday tasks. This critical self-reflection enables physicians to listen attentively to patients' distress, recognize their own errors, refine their technical skills, make evidence-based decisions, and clarify their values so that they can act with compassion, technical competence, presence, and insight.[29]

Healing Intentions

The concept of intention has become an interesting inquiry within the field of consciousness studies. Ordinary clinical work deals with *objective* consciousness, discovered in patients through physical or mental state examinations.[30] However, within a person's general *subjective* consciousness (wakefulness), awareness includes a diffused external environment, as a background screen upon which one may direct *attention* to some specific object or task; *intention* introduces a special sense of connectedness to that object (an object of thought, perhaps). In its ordinary meaning, intention indicates a will to cause an effect (though the question of how "free" can free-will be is a tangled subject all its own[31]). Within the context of theories of quantum mind, a state of intention infers connectedness to the (nonlocal) unconscious mind. Remote effects, such as the researcher-effect and prayer-effect mentioned earlier, imply that there may also be an efficacious connectedness to the quantum nonlocality, wherein all effects are mediated.

In 1988, Byrd[32] divided patients admitted to a coronary-care unit into a control group (no special intervention) and a group which was prayed for by strangers at a remote location, unbeknownst to the patients and staff. Harris *et al.*[33] replicated the study, except that their scoring system was somewhat different. Both studies showed fewer complications in the prayer groups (at borderline significance levels), though not differences in survival. Krucoff *et al.*[34] showed a statistically significant reduction in complications in prayed-for patients undergoing percutaneous coronary interventions. Schlitz and Braud,[35] Astin *et al.*[36], and Dossey[37] have reviewed various studies (of human and non-human systems) of distant-intentionality, showing a positive effect in many studies, but not all.

Prompted by such results, Benson *et al*[38] undertook a much larger study in six hospitals in the United States. Patients about to undergo coronary artery bypass surgery were randomized into three groups (enrollment 1998-2000). Patients in one group were informed that they might or might not be prayed for (by off-site groups of various faith perspectives). A second group was informed that they would be prayed for. Results were analyzed according to expectations of receiving prayer:

(a) those uncertain whether they would be prayed for, but who did receive prayer (n=604);

(b) those uncertain, who were not prayed for by a study prayer group (n=597);

(c) those who knew before surgery that they were in the group to be prayed for (n=601).

Results were calculated according to complication rates, major and minor. There was no apparent effect of being prayed for in the (a) vs. (b) groups. However, those in (c), who knew before surgery that they were assigned to the group to be prayed-for, had a higher general complication rate than patients in (a) who received prayer but did not know their status as to prayer. Major complications, including 30-day mortality rates, were reported as similar in all the groups.

The study design, of "certain" vs. "uncertain" was intended to address the major hidden variable in any prayer study involving illness. It is very likely that most people in hospital in the United States are prayed for (or are at least the object of *special healing intentions)* by someone in their personal environment, regardless of the patient's own faith perspective, whether or not a study is in progress. Study of a large number of patients hopes to average out that problem, but making the calculation of a definitive study size requires at least estimating the size of this variable. It is also unknown what proportion of the population is "susceptible" (sensitive) to nonlocal effects, thus (presumably) being more likely to respond to prayerful intentions.

In view of the above discussion on noetic effects in general, one may cite several other possibly confounding effects for studies of this type. For a multicenter study it becomes especially hard to control for variables such as investigator skepticism (or lack of it), and the general "placebo effects" of staff personality and "atmosphere" of caring in the respective institutions. A particularly difficult issue is how to approach

those patients in (c). It would be very hard indeed to inform
the six hundred scattered among six institutions over a two
year period, without leaving an implication in at least some
of them that "the Hospital" has put them in a special group,
so "it must be worse than I thought".[38a]

That of course is a purely conjectural comment, intended only
to highlight formidable difficulties in establishing nonlocal
effects, especially among patients undergoing technically
elaborate interventions. The positive (but weak) effects of
prayer reported earlier were generally in patients having
no or (relatively) minor procedures in a medical, not major-
surgical context. At the very least we now have learned that
"officially" telling patients of assignment to a prayer group is
probably not good medicine, at least not unless a very carefully screened patient indicates that it would be welcome.
There is another concern: the effect in question is a nonlocal effect. If there are such effects why might they not occur
among staff as well? If so, rules regarding blinding of staff to
patients' study status would not necessarily protect against
subtle "noetic cues". The principles of study design, so well
established for physical studies, may well require modifica-
tion when studying nonlocal effects.

In other studies, prayer had no effect in treatment of alcohol
abuse,[39] or in psychological or rheumatic disease. O'Laoire[41]
studied psychological measures of normal volunteers who
were prayed for. In that study, agents (who prayed) scored
better than subjects (those prayed for), but both groups showed
a statistically significant prayer effect. For the agents, more

prayer correlated with more improvement in the agents' own scores. (O'Laoire also made the interesting but untested suggestion that the greater the strain within the organism—the offset from homeostatic balance—the greater the potential for response to prayer.)

The reported effects of prayer clearly lie outside normal biomedical expectations. Koenig and others,[42] who have reviewed 1200 epidemiological studies correlating religion and health,[43] noted their skepticism about prayer studies which supposedly derive from mechanisms "for which there is no scientific explanation." By contrast, the benefits of the reported epidemiological studies can be "understood in terms of well-known and established psychosocial, behavioral, and biological pathways."

The review by Astin *et al.* of "distant healing" also showed effect in some (separately tabulated) studies of *Therapeutic Touch*. However, therapeutic touch is not nonlocal in the reality sense. Any effect might easily be interpreted as an effect of normal consciousness, since the presence and proximity of the therapist are known to the patient, even though the therapist tries not touch the patient physically.

Many medical centers and healthcare groups are responding to increased patient interest in alternative and complementary approaches to personal health. Too often, however, the new programs function relatively independently, under a philosophy not widely shared among the medical staff. If most patients are self-referred, any benefit achieved may remain unrecognized by the patient's (perhaps skeptic) physicians, a situation especially likely when the programs are initiated by the administration for "market" reasons. Integration of medical/surgical care and mind/spirit care awaits a noetic approach, namely, a truly unitive philosophy of caring shared by all involved: patients, physicians, allied health personnel, administration, *and* payers.

In an attempt to introduce his breast cancer patients (and others) to the benefits of conscious, *intentional* participation in personal healing, the author developed a pilot program called *Healing Intentions*.[44] The program invited patients to participate at whatever level felt comfortable, in small groups which blended mindfulness meditation with dialog about life-stress management and healing as an individualized process of restoring balance to life. *Medical intentions* emphasized Benson's relaxation response with particular attention to physiological benefits. *Psychological intentions* introduced guided imagery, the idea of cognitive health, and recognition of the personal unconscious. *Spiritual intentions* invited extended mindfulness meditation (contemplative or centering prayer) for the experience of the spiritual ("eternal," nonlocal) realm.

The outline of the program recognizes that patients need (and perhaps, want) certain levels of personal involvement at different stages of illness. Consider as a generic example, the patient who discovers a breast lump. The immediate adjunctive need (*medical intention*) is for stress-management while the diagnosis is established, and cognitive learning and assent as she deals with decisions about further therapy. Specific psychological problems might prompt mental health consultations, but it is during followup chemotherapy or radiotherapy that guided imagery and psychosocial support (*psychological intentions*) might become especially helpful. *Spiritual intentions* become more important as the patient "picks up the pieces" to reestablish an ordered life with a new sense of meaning and purpose, not merely *coping* with the illness, but triumphantly *transcending* it, perhaps even in the face of advanced disease.

Medical Spirituality

Patients with a developed spiritual or religious sense often express a concern that most modern medicine is hostile, or at least insensitive, to the soul aspect of life. Whether or not they have a developed religious sense, patients often present with a sense of spiritual "emptiness", especially at times of confronting major surgery or grave disease. Of course, "emptiness" is not a clinical diagnosis, and such patients do not want referral to a psychiatrist.

The obvious place for such patients to turn is to a trusted member of the clergy; but for many patients in our society, there is no such relationship. Many have abandoned traditional faith because of difficulty in believing what literalist traditions require them to believe; and many others have rejected, or been rejected by, their traditional faiths for reasons of lifestyle, such as non-traditional family structures.

Unspoken spiritual problems are often a factor in non-compliance with recommended clinical treatments, or in seeking unconventional therapies. Sometimes, such concerns may not become evident until they become overt illness (e.g. somatization, stress syndromes, or depression), or social pathology (e.g. violent behavior and victimization of others). Both categories of problem have substantially increased in society during the three decades in which I have been in surgical practice.

If we as physicians individually, or as a profession, are truly to offer a return to health and well-being to such patients, we must develop an appropriate concept and language for discussing such abstractions as "spiritual emptiness" during a medical encounter, and prepare ourselves to deal with the patients' responses.

Sloan *et al.*[45] have taken strong exception to incorporating spirituality concerns into medical practice. Koenig *et al.*[46] replied to the substantive arguments, but in reply to correspondence, Sloan[47] acknowledges that turf issues also are a concern. Indeed, many disciplines contribute to knowledge about the complex relationships between health and spirituality, and each would thus have some claim to "turf".

Bessinger and Kuhne[48] proposed that presently there is sufficient weight of information to justify defining *medical spirituality* as a distinct interdisciplinary field of interest within medical and allied health practice. Such a designation could help define the domains and boundaries for appropriate cooperative clinical practice and research, consistent with the evidence-based approach; help integrate the new perspective on nonlocality; and help preempt developing turf issues.

The current literature offers no consensus about definitions for *religion* or *spirituality*. The following definitions offered by Bessinger and Kuhne provide a distinction which makes it easier to interpret new research findings, and distinguish levels of appropriate physician involvement in patient's spiritual concerns.

Spirituality is the personal function which relates life's meaning to transpersonal reality. *Spirituality* is an element of a person's individuality, and is not necessarily defined by association with a certain tradition or by organizational affiliation. It is multidimensional, and operates (to varying degrees) in acknowledgment of the unconscious self, of the needs of others, and of the realm of the sacred. Such awareness varies among individuals and throughout a person's lifetime. Waldfogel[49] has summarized the elements of spirituality as they relate to medical practice. *Transpersonal reality* here refers to those levels of *world* beyond the ordinary bounds of ego-consciousness. It includes the level of *transcendence* as used by Waldfogel, and Cassell.[50]

Religion refers to the set of beliefs and practices shared by a community in reaching toward the transpersonal reality. This also is a broad term, but describes a more collective element. Each *religion* has its own historical tradition with a rich and complex symbolic language by which to interpret its central symbol of the deepest level of transpersonal reality. Such language may easily be misunderstood by people outside the tradition.

Medical spirituality, as a domain of special clinical interest, education, and research within the healthcare field, would encompass (1) the clinical basis of knowledge and skill by which to assess and respond to patient needs; (2) the philosophic basis for noetic practice, such as is attempted in the present study; (3) professional activities designed to encourage practitioners with non-sectarian peer support and personal development; and (4) studies of the ethical, legal, and social implications of the field of practice. A special ethical concern is that practitioners restrict themselves to doing what they do well, develop effective networks with colleagues, and make appropriate referrals. Another is that the skills and knowledge of medical spirituality serve the purposes of healing practice, rather than the advancement of sectarian agendas zealously pursued.

Medical Intuition

"The whole art of medicine is in observation."[51] That already old maxim was taken by Sir William Osler as a summary of his method of teaching. He also wrote, "The value of experience is not in seeing much, but in seeing wisely," and "Observation *plus* thinking has given us the vast stores of knowledge we now possess ...".

But what are we to observe? In our conventional approach to medical practice, the object of our observation is that described by Osler as "the book of Nature written large in the bodies of men." Now, the further unfolding of that book of Nature is written even larger and in much more detail. It includes knowledge of both body and mind, the very mind which engages, and is engaged by, Nature as object and subject.

The individual mind has a variety of functions involved in its observing process. We have noted them in Part III, as the *complementarities* of sensing-intuition by which information is received, and thinking-valuing (or feeling) by which information is weighed. Clearly, modern medical practice (and science generally) functions in the sensing and thinking modes, and typically pays little notice to the intuition and valuing aspects of mental operation. That situation determines, and is determined by, our prevailing mechanistic worldview. In noetic practice, the physician's own mind becomes a valued object of observation, through the practice called mindfulness. Preserving the valuable sensing-thinking faculties while bringing them into their proper complementary relationship with intuition and valuing "tunes the mind" into a proper instrument of medical art.

Neil Prose[52] offered a helpful example in JAMA's occasional feature, "A Piece of my Mind." He was discussing with a medical student an ordinary encounter in the clinic. The student mentioned seeing a momentary tear on the youth's face during the interview. The attending returned to the room for a private discussion with the patient, and learned of deep concerns which otherwise would not have been recognized, and which were the key to understanding the teen's problem. In that situation, the student exemplifies the natural use of the intuition-feeling modes which so often seem to become dessicated during our medical training.

Undoubtedly most of us who have been in practice long enough have come across clinical situations in which a "gut feeling" made an important difference. I know of a patient who went to a surgeon to see about a painfully ingrown toenail. The surgeon ordered a CT scan of the head and found a meningioma. (Fortunately that was in the days before managed care.) The key was in the *way* he listened to her complaint, noting an element of disorganization and confusion, which was new for her. In another situation, a radiologist who prided himself on mastery of the points of mammographic diagnosis, wrote that the calcifications clearly were benign and no further workup was indicated. However, a surgeon (who had contact with the patient) saw the same films but had a different *feeling* about them; the biopsy showed carcinoma-in-situ.

Of course, such tales are "merely anecdotes" but of course, all *experience* is anecdotal, and all experience is mental and subjective, not objective. Nor is knowledge of a probability distribution much help in confronting an individual patient. It is only by careful observations using both sensing and intuiting abilities, and by careful evaluation using both thinking and valuing (feeling) abilities, that we "collapse the wave function" of the presenting probabilities. Only thus do we determine whether the patient before us is the one exception in the cohort of a hundred similar cases.

Quantum mind theories have opened up new avenues for understanding the personal relationship between mind and the nonlocal and probabilistic cosmos, whose inherent logic is complementarity. Deep intuition seems somehow to involve a direct connection to or correlation with the nonlocal connecting principle.

As such, it could be a process for reading the wisdom inherent in the connectedness of a situation, to which we may profitably listen. How do we cultivate it? Mindfulness practice can cultivate it, insofar as intuition is an aspect of mindfulness, as can perhaps developing sensitivities for creativity and art. Thankfully, we can learn to trust our own intuitions, but claims of self-described "medical intuitives" have been notoriously difficult, if not impossible, to corroborate.

Even though results so far have varied widely, we now can glimpse, as if across a threshold, exciting possibilities of using mental power in new ways to influence healing through intention and intuition. Schlitz[53] has reminded us that we do not yet know whether intuition can always be corroborated by conventional sensing techniques. New kinds of research techniques may be required. Indeed, new types of studies are already being developed, for it is on evidence we must rely, even as we move more deeply into the noetic world. After all, that is the world we live in, the world which awaits the further blossoming of healing thought.

An Afterword

It has been a recurring dream for several years, but with many variations. No, not the surgeon's classic nightmare of instruments which don't work, of uncontrolled bleeding, or of endlessly frustrating breaks in aseptic technique, or awful internal deformities defying repair. But the dream usually leaves me with an unsettled feeling, nonetheless.

I am in a hospital, sometimes my medical school hospital, or the building (now razed) where I did surgical training. It is usually undergoing some sort of renovation, and I am having difficulty getting to my patients. Perhaps it is a blocked stairwell, or the stairwell does not lead to where I want to go. Or an ancient elevator cab gets stuck, or the wrong end opens. Or it doesn't stop on my floor.

In one variation, I cannot get into my hall locker (why hall lockers as in high school?) but the (female) head nurse comes and brings the key. In another, the rickety elevator in the oldest part of the building discharges me onto a gutted upper floor. All partitions have been removed, for new ones are being constructed. Heavy cables lie loosely on the floor. A workman warns me to watch out especially for the end of the large one nearest me, for it carries high voltage.

Another time, I am trying to find my way to the cafeteria of my medical school hospital, and find myself in a newly opened and disconcertingly modernistic lobby.

Whatever the personal meanings for me (and I still ponder them in retirement), the dreams seem also to have a collective aspect, offering images that tell a story about the dilemma which so many of us in medicine express today.

Clearly the house of healing is undergoing substantial renovations, and most of us, physicians, other staff, and patients alike, feel a great sense of disquiet. Patients often respond by seeking "alternative" healthcare. Physicians increasingly are opting out too, taking the *alternative* of early retirement. At the same time, there are signs that the megaconglomerate managed care corporations are feeling the strain too, and that a reorganization of all our arrangements and attitudes within healthcare is immanent. But where will the new partitions go? And how is that high-voltage cable to be connected?

The current view of nonlocality points to a powerful new concept of health, which ultimately is grounded within its deepest processes of consciousness. Noetic practice affords the medical profession the possibility of touching that most basic level of human health much more deeply, and opens up a wide range of new possibilities for helping, in disease and in health.

This is not merely a peripheral or optional concern, for now there is evidence that struggles of the spirit can literally make a difference between life and death. Pargament *et al.* [1] report a two-year longitudinal study of elderly patients admitted for medical illness, in which higher scores of religious struggle (or "spiritual discontent") predicted greater risk of mortality.

Clearly such data indicate both opportunity and imperative. A reconciliation of medical philosophy with physical and clinical evidence will be necessary if we are to develop the full potential of noetic practice. May it also provide a renewed sense of meaning and purpose to all who practice now and those who will come after, who reach out to heal ...

It is the most comprehensive job on earth,
because it means caring for the complete human being
— not just the body.

It means sympathy with human suffering,
understanding of human despair,
knowledge of human weakness
— and the power of helping. [2]

Notes and References

References ordinarily acknowledge sources to help buttress the ideas presented. However, in a multi-disciplinary work such as this, perhaps they are even more important as a guide toward further study of topics of special interest. Many original sources are cited, but also summaries written by experts for a general, university level readership. Since some entries have several elements, all notes, comments, internet citations, and references to printed work are placed here. Full citations of printed works are placed in the bibliography.

Part I : A Medical Reality Check

1. Nadeau & Kafatos; Herbert; Baggott; Aspect (1982; 2007); Groeblacher. Experimental support of nonlocal reality has grown stronger since confirmed by Aspect, 1982. Studies of quantum computing also confirm various aspects of *entanglement* of correlated photons, a nonlocal property on which quantum computing depends, and several recent studies have now shown entanglement occurring in atomic systems; i.e. quantum effects can be seen within the realm previously called *classical*. For example, see Ginsberg NS et al; Fleischhauer; Jost JD *et al.*; Blatt R.; Schlosshauer; Ball. Thus it is appropriate to look for nonlocal effects (such as synchronicities, complementarities, etc.) in the ordinary phenomenal world of consciousness.

2. Herbert, p. 242

3. Hawking, 2001; Smolin, 1997, pp. 79-80

4. Kaku; Greene

5. Baggott

6. Zurek, 1991

7. Baggott

8. Zurek, 2001; Zewail

9. Gleick; Briggs; Albrecht

10. Gleick; Briggs; Whitfield; Ben-Jacob and Levine

11. Penrose, 1994; Nadeau and Kafatos, p. 174

12. Hameroff; Hameroff & Penrose

13. Sheldrake (1981), rev. 1995, appendix pp.221-222

14. Denton & Marshall; Kirschner *et al.* Also, Taylor (2002) re protein folding as being guided by a mathematical grammar of ideal structures, or "Forms" (Taylor's quotation marks presumably allude to Plato).

15. Hawking, 1988

16. Hawking, 1988; Barrow & Tipler

17. Jung, 1968

18. Jung *et al.*, 1964; Campbell 1974

19. Jung, 1968; Stevens; Edinger

20. Jung, 1969; Peat.

20a. The Global Consciousness Project: see http://noosphere. princeton.edu/ . (Accessed June 2009).

21. Byrd; Harris *et al.*; Schlitz & Braud; Krucoff *et al.*; Astin *et al.*; Benson H. *et al.* (2006). See further discussion in Parts III, IV.

22. Bertalanffy. The material remaining in Part I is adapted from Bessinger, 1996.

23. Herbert; Barrow & Tipler; Baggott

24. Hawking, 1988

25. Barrow & Tipler

26. Bergson; Whitehead

27. Teilhard, 1975, pp.64-65. Note especially Teilhard's idea that "essentially all energy is psychic in nature."

28. Lederman; Veltman

29. Lederman, p. 376

30. Greene; Hawking 2001; Smolin 2001

31. Smolin, 2001. See also Penrose, 1989; Barrow, 1991

32. Penrose R quoted by Horgan

33. Baggott; Barrow & Tipler; Goswami, 1993

34. Jung, 1968; and see Edinger; Stevens; Nunn, 1998; Atmanspacher, 1998

35. Jung, 1969; Peat

36. Atmanspacher & Primas; Peat

37. Davies

38. Greene

39. One of the theories which seeks to explain the "quantum reality" invokes a concept of "many worlds," that is, many universes existing simultaneously (Everett and Wheeler, see Herbert; Hawking, 2001). Another (Smolin, 1997) proposes evolution and natural selection of universes, of which this one just happens to contain consciousness. For simplicity's sake, we will discuss our one visible universe in relationship to the reality-dimensions which nurture it. Conceptually, that reality may include other universes, but they would be beyond our reach, and could contribute nothing helpful to our discussion. Further, if the speculation about pulsed nonlocality is correct, the nonlocality would itself be a "multiverse" of probabilities being resolved at each plick, into one instantaneous actuality.

40. Shear

41. Goswami, 1993

42. That is, a unit of thought (an abstract concept), described from a spacetime point of view. Language fails, when one tries to speak of "units" in a realm which knows no boundary. To an observer in the nuocontinuum, all points in spacetime would be seen as one; the life of the universe would have no history or beginning, but would be experienced only as a present-tense steady state (if there could be any *experience* at all, in the absence of a time-reference). The creative "thought" or process of the universe extends its logic in a non-temporal realm (cf. Whitehead).

42a. See Barbour re distinction between Schrödinger's time-dependent and time-independent equations.

43. Hawking quoted by Barrow & Tipler, p. 458.

Part II : The Nature of Nonlocal Reality

1. Roukes; Feynman, 1959. "All the way down" recalls an amusing story by Hawking (1988, p. 1), about turtles.

2. Aspect; Herbert, p. 226-227; Baggott, p. 139-150; Rowe

3. Bohm, 1983

4. Bohm & Hiley, 1993

5. Bohm & Hiley, 1993, p. 37-38

6. Bohm & Hiley, 1993, p. 57

7. Zurek, 1991

8. Zurek, 2001; Albrecht

9. Goswami, 1993, 1994

10. Atmanspacher & Primas

11. Sheldrake, 1988, p.109

12. Sheldrake, 1988, p. 97

13. Sheldrake, 1988, p.109. Sheldrake (*Psych.Persp.* 1987, 1988) has also related morphic resonance to Jung's archetypal theory. Archetypes are special "habits of nature." The nuocontinuum theory would explain them as patterns of psychic experience nonlocally integrated throughout human history, which is basically the same concept.

14. The report of scoring beauty in composite photographs is based on a November 1996 broadcast of "Discovery magazine" (Discovery channel) reporting research by a Harvard neuropsychologist, Nancy Etcoff. Her idea came from a nineteenth century series of blended mug shots. The result was not the sought for "criminal characteristics," but handsome faces. I have been unable to retrieve a journal reference.

15. Hameroff & Penrose, 1996

16. Hameroff & Penrose, 1996, p.36

17. Hameroff & Penrose, 1996, p.37

18. Penrose, 1989, p. 429

19. Smolin, 1997

20. Clarke

20a. Barbour. His imagery of a "blue mist" of superposed quantum potentialities, declaring itself as "red" or "green" at each instant, seems especially helpful in visualizing the stream of interchanges between local and nonlocal aspects of reality.

21. We will be working here with the standard model of quantum physics, which is most easily expressed in terms of Schrödinger's probabilistic equation. The evolution of emphasis in quantum theory toward information exchanges (as predicted by Smolin, 2001) would seem to strengthen the case for the time-based interim theory developed here. The probabilities referred to in the discussion can be understood as derived from more fundamental information exchanges within nonlocality. That would also accord with the rapidly developing field of quantum computing, which is also of increasing interest for quantum mind approaches to consciousness. For a view of cosmos as computational, see Lloyd.

22. Lykken.

23. Kaku

24. Whitehead

25. Campbell, 1983

26. Bergson; Whitehead

27. tr. Bly

27a. Cellular automata are entertaining examples of creation by iteration. See Wolfram.

28. Penrose, 1994; Byron & Fuller

29. Bohm

30. Bohm and Hiley

31. Feynman, 1948; Penrose, 1994

32. Zurek, 1991

33. Hawking & Penrose

34. Smolin, 1997; Greene

35. Hawking & Penrose, p 65

36. Penrose, 1994; Hameroff, 1994; Hameroff & Penrose, 1996

37. Jibu, Pribham KH, & Yasue ; Pribham; Globus. For general comment on theories of quantum mind, see Esfeld; Nunn 1994; Squires; Stapp

38. *Potentia* is Heisenberg's term for the probabilistic precursor states of quantum actualities (see Herbert).

39. A quality which the author has shamelessly exploited in his *Poetic Works*, 2009

Part III. Healing Thought

1. Bessinger, 1988.

2. Glick; Bessinger, 1988

3. For example, Figure 1 in the report by Singletary on breast carcinogenesis.

4. Bertalanffy

5. Engle.

6. Nadeau and Kafatos, especially pp. 100-103

7. Jung, 1923.

8. These personality types are tested by the Meyers-Briggs Personality Inventory, which also scores whether the "rational" set (*judging* type) or the "non-rational" set (*perceiving* type) is the stronger. These types are designated by initials, such as INTJ or ESFP. There are sixteen possible combinations.

9. Cannon

10. Wilber, 1995, Chapter 2

11. *Nuoflux* is a new word, contrived to suggest that the nuocontinuum has its dynamic process, even though it is difficult to visualize and describe with spacetime language and imagery.

12. Wang *et al.* re gastric motility; Makikallio *et al.*, Vikman *et al.*, and Clayton and Murray re arrhythmia; see also, Yeragani *et al.* on cardiac rhythm nonlinearity and panic disorder.

13. Kahn *et al.*

14. Frenkel and Hermoni; Linde *et al.*

15. Wiseman and Schlitz

16. Rosa *et al.*

17. Astin *et al.*

18. Roberts *et al.*

19. Targ

20. These concepts are adapted from a table by Fontanarosa and Lundberg.

Part IV. Noetic Practice

1. Krizek

2. Schweitzer, selected by Cousins. Part IV draws heavily on Bessinger, 1993, also available at http://home.earthlink.net/~dbscr/Medsoul.htm (Accessed February 2009; case sensitive)

3. Moore

4. Jung, 1933

5. Michels and Marzuk

6. Folkman

7. Garg

8. Kiecolt-Glasser *et al.*, 2001

9. Hiramoto *et al.*; Miller *et al.*

10. Kiecolt-Glasser *et al.*, 1998

11. Dantzer

12. Miller *et al.*

13. Anderson

14. Petrie

15. Spiegel *et al.*, 1989; Spiegel, 1999

16. Greer

17. Wickramasekera (and see extensive bibliography and related articles in the same issue of *Advances*)

18. O'Regan and Hirshberg

19. Wiseman and Schlitz

20. Skelly

21. Cassell, 1976, pp 136-138

22. Waldfogel

23. "Health Yourself" (2002). Dean Health System, Madison, WI 53713

24. Murphy and Donovan; Benson

25. Hayward

26. Keating describes a Christian approach.

27. Benson

28. Kabat-Zinn *et al.*, 1986; Kabat-Zinn, 1991, 1994

29. Epstein

30. See Petty for a neurosurgical perspective.

31. Consider the 1983 Libet experiments, in which subjects marked the first moment of awareness of intent to move, which occurred only after the appearance of the action potential of the movement within the motor cortex. (Haggard and Libet, 2001)

32. Byrd *et al.*

33. Harris *et al.*

34. Krucoff *et al.*

35. Schlitz and Braud

36. Astin *et al.*

37. Dossey

38. Benson *et al.*, 2006

38a. One might well recall that in certain strict religious traditions, "I'll pray for you" can have a heavily-loaded judgmental connotation.

39. Walker *et al.*

40. Joyce and Welldon

41. O'Laoire.

42. Koenig *et al.*, 1999

43. Koenig *et al.*, 2001

44. See Bessinger, 1997, http:/home.earthlink.net/~dbscr/aih/ hi-ms.htm (accessed June 2009, case-sensitive)—a summary prepared for patients. The program was tried in three venues, with considerable patient appreciation and interest, but formidable problems (physician factors, funding, etc.) defeated establishment of a continuation program. Nevertheless, the outline may be helpful to others in devising similar efforts in other communities. (Creative Commons License: http://creativecommons. org/licenses/by-nc-sa/3.0/) In today's market, establishing such a program would require the continuity offered by institutional sponsorship and staffing; and philanthropic funding.

45. Sloan *et al.*, 1999; Sloan *et al.*, 2000 (June)

46. Koenig *et al.*, 1999

47. Sloan *et al.*, 2000 (Nov)

48. Bessinger and Kuhne, 2002

49. Waldfogel

50. Cassell, 1982

51. Sir William Osler (1849-1919), quoted by Bryan, pp. 109-112

52. Prose

53. Schlitz, 2002

An Afterword

1. Pargament *et al.*

2. Anonymous, an inscription by a friend in the author's pre-med yearbook, 1957.

This monograph brings together material from other articles by the author, published (as cited) and unpublished (but previously posted on the internet). Draft version completed 2002. Revised and updated June 2009.

Bibliography

Albrecht A Quantum ripples in chaos. *Nature,* 2001 (16 Aug); 412: 687-688

Anderson JL. The immune system and major depression. *Advances in Neuroimmunology,* 1996; 6:119-129

Aspect A, Dalibard J. Experimental test of Bell's inequalities using time-varying analyzers. *Phys. Rev. Lett.* 1982: 49, 1804-1807

Aspect A. Bell's inequality test: more ideal than ever. *Nature,* 1999 (Mar 18); 398: 189-190.

Aspect A. Quantum mechanics: To be or not to be local. *Nature,* 2007 (19 April); 446: 866-867

Astin JA, Harkness E, Ernst E. The efficacy of "distant healing": A systematic review of randomized trials. *Annals of Internal Medicine,* 2000: 132: 903-910.

Atmanspacher H. Commentary on Chris Nunn's 'Archetypes and memes'. *J. Consc. Studies,* 1998 ; 5: 355-361

Atmanspacher H and Primas H. The hidden side of Wolfgang Pauli. *Journal of Consciousness Studies,* 1996; 3(2): 112-126.

Baggott J. *The Meaning of Quantum Theory.* New York: Oxford University Press, 1992.

Ball P. Physics: Quantum all the way. *Nature,* 2008: 453, 22-25

Barbour J. *The End of Time: The Next Revolution in Physics.* Oxford University Press, 1999.

Barrow JD. *Theories of Everything: The Quest for Ultimate Explanation,*New York: Oxford/Clarendon Press, 1991

Barrow JD and Tipler FJ. *The Anthropic Cosmological Principle.* Oxford: Oxford U. Press, 1986:463

Ben-Jacob E, Levine H. The artistry of nature. *Nature,* 2001 (22 Feb); 409: 985-986.

Benson H. *The Relaxation Response.* New York: Avon Books, 1976.

Benson H *et al.* Study of the Therapeutic Effects of Intercessory Prayer (STEP) in cardiac bypass patients: a multicenter randomized trial of uncertainty and certainty of receiving intercessory prayer. *Am Heart J,* 2006; 151(4): 934-942.

Bergson H. *Creative Evolution.* New York: Henry Holt, 1911

Bertalanffy L. *General Systems Theory: Foundations, Development, Applications.* New York: Braziler, 1968

Bessinger D. Doctoring: The Philosophic Milieu. *Southern Med J.* 1988, December. 81: 1558-1562.

Bessinger D. *Poetic Works,* BookSurge Publishing, 2009

Bessinger D. Reflections on "soul" and medical art. *Journal of the SC Medical Association,* 1993 (Dec); 89:572-575.

Bessinger D. Reflections on reality, healing and consciousness. *Alternative Therapies in Health and Medicine,* 1996; 2(2): 40-45.

Bessinger D and Kuhne T. Medical spirituality: defining domains and boundaries. *Southern Medical Journal,* 2002 (Dec); 95:1385-1388

Blatt, R. Entanglement goes mechanical. *Nature,* 2009 (4 June); 459:653-654

Bly R. *The Soul is Here for Its Own Joy.* Hopewell NJ: Ecco Press, 1995, p. 88.

Bohm D. *Wholeness and the Implicate Order.* New York: Arc/Routledge & Kegan Paul, 1983

Bohm D, Hiley BJ. *The Undivided Universe: An Ontological Interpretation of Quantum Theory .* New York: Routledge, 1993

Briggs J. *Fractals, the Patterns of Chaos.* New York: Simon & Schuster, 1992.

Bryan CS. *Osler, Inspirations from a Great Physician.* Oxford University Press, 1997

Byrd RC. Positive therapeutic effects of intercessory prayer in a coronary care unit population. *Southern Medical Journal,* 1988; 81(7):826-829. Reprint: *Alternative Therapies in Health and Medicine,* 1997; 3(6): 87-90.

Byron FW, Fuller RW. *Mathematics of Classical and Quantum Physics.* Mineola NY: Dover, 1992

Campbell J (ed.) *Man and Time: Papers from the Eranos Yearbooks* (1957), Princeton NJ: Princeton University Press, Bollingen Series, 1983

Campbell J. *The Mythic Image.* Princeton University Press, 1974.

Cannon W. Organization for physiological homeostasis. *Physiological Reviews* 1929; 9: 399-431.

Cassell EJ. The nature of suffering and the goals of medicine. *N Engl J Med,* 1982; 306: 639-645.

Cassell EJ. *The Healer's Art* (1976). MIT Press, 1985.

Clarke CJS. The nonlocality of mind, *Journal of Consciousness Studies,* 1995; 2(3): 231-240.

Clayton RH, Murray A. Linear and non-linear analysis of the surface electrocardiogram during human ventricular fibrillation shows evidence of order in the underlying mechanism. *Medical & Biological Engineering and Computing,* 1999 (May); 37: 354-358

Dantzer R. Stress and immunity: what have we learned from psychoneuroimmunology? *Acta Physiol Scand Suppl,* 1997; 640: 43-46

Davies, P. *Superforce: The Search for a Grand Unified Theory of Nature.* New York: Simon and Schuster, 1985:152 ff.

Denton M, Marshall C. Laws of form revisited. *Nature,* 2001 (Mar 22); 410: 417

Dossey L. *Healing Words: The Power of Prayer and the Practice of Medicine.* HarperSanFrancisco, 1993.

Edinger E. *Ego and Archetype.* Boston: Shambhala, 1992.

Engel GL. The need for a new medical model: A challenge for biomedicine. *Science* 1977; 196:129-36

Epstein RM. Mindful practice. *J Amer Med Assoc.* 1999 (Sep 1); 282: 833-839. (104 refs.)

Esfeld M. Quantum holism and the philosophy of mind. *J Consc Studies,* 1999; 6: 23-38

Feynman RP. There's plenty of room at the bottom (lecture, 1959). http://www.its.caltech.edu/~feynman (accessed June 2009)

Feynman RP. Space-time approach to non-relativistic quantum mechanics, *Reviews in Modern Physics,* 1948; 20:367-387. Cited by Penrose 1994

Fleischauer M. Quantum physics: Indistinguishable from afar. *Nature* 445, 605-606 (8 February 2007)

Folkman S. Thoughts about psychological factors, PNI, and cancer. *Advances in Mind-Body Medicine,* 1999; 15: 255-259.

Fontanarosa PB and Lundberg GD. Alternative medicine meets science (editorial). *Journal of the American Medical Association,* 1998 (Nov 11); 280-1618-1619.

Frenkel M, Hermoni D. Effects of homeopathic intervention of medication consumption in atopic and allergic disorders. *Alternative Therapies in Health and Medicine,* 2002; 8: 76-79.

Garg A *et al.* Psychological stress perturbs epidermal permeability barrier homeostasis: Implications for the pathogenesis of stress-associated skin disorders. *Archives of Dermatology,* 2001; 137: 53-59

Ginsberg NS, Garner SR & Hau LV. Coherent control of optical information with matter wave dynamics. *Nature* 445, 623–626 (2007),

Gleick J. *Chaos: Making a new science.* Penguin Books, 1988

Glick SM. Humanistic medicine in a modern age. *N Eng J Med* 1981; 304: 1036-38.

Globus G. Self, cognition, qualia and world in quantum brain dynamics. *J Consc Studies,* 1998; 5(1): 34-52.

Goswami A. *The Self-Aware Universe: How Consciousness Creates the Material World,* New York: Tarcher/Putnam, 1993:78-97

Goswami A. *Science Within Consciousness: Developing a Science Based on the Primacy of Consciousness.* Petaluma CA: Institute of Noetic Sciences, Research Report (Causality Project CP- 7), 1994.

Greene B. *The Elegant Universe.* New York: Vintage Books/Random House, 1999.

Greer S. Mind-body research in psychooncology. *Advances in Mind-Body Medicine,* 1999; 15: 236-244

Groeblacher S *et al.* An experimental test of non-local realism *Nature,* 2007 (19 April); 446: 871-875.

Haggard P and Libet B. Conscious intention and brain activity. *J. Consc. Studies,* 2001 ; 8: 47-63

Hameroff S and Penrose R. Conscious events as orchestrated space-time selections. *Journal of Consciousness Studies,* 1996; 3(1):36-53

Hameroff SA. Quantum coherence in microtubules: A neural basis for emergent consciousness? *J Consc Studies,* 1994; 1(1): 91-118

Harris WS, Gowda M, Kolb JW *et al.* A randomized controlled trial of the effects of remote intercessory prayer on outcomes in patients admitted to the coronary care unit. *Archives of Internal Medicine,* 1999; 159(19): 2273-2278.

Hawking SW. *A Brief History of Time from the Big Bang to Black Holes.* New York: Bantam, 1988:174

Hawking SW, Penrose R. *The Nature of Space and Time.* Princeton NJ: Princeton University Press, 1995

Hawking, SW. *The Universe in a Nutshell.* New York: Bantam, 2001.

Hayward J. A rDzogs-chen interpretation of the sense of self. *J Cons Studies,* 1998; 5: 611-626

Herbert N. *Quantum Reality: Beyond the New Physics.* Garden City NY: Anchor/ Doubleday, 1985

Hiramoto RN *et al.* Psychoneuroendocrine immunology: perception of stress can alter body termperature and natural killer cell activity. *International Journal of Neuroscience,* 1999; 98: 95-129 (Review, 127 refs)

Horgan J. Particle Metaphysics. *Scientific American* 1994 (Feb); 270(2):96-106

Jibu M, Pribham KH, Yasue K. From conscious experience to memory storage and retrieval: The role of quantum brain dynamics and boson condensation of evanescent photons. *Int J Mod Physics B,* 1996;10:1735-54. Cited by Pribham KH. 1999

Jost JD *et al.* Entangled mechanical oscillators. *Nature,* 2009 (4 June); 459:683-685.

Joyce CR, Welldon RM. The objective efficacy of prayer: a double-blind clinical trial. *J Chronic Dis.,* 1965; 18: 367-377 (cited by Astin *et al.*)

Jung CG. *Psychological Types: General Description of the Types* (1923) . Collected Works 6.; Princeton U. Press/Bollingen.

Jung CG. *Modern Man in Search of a Soul* (1933). Harcourt Brace Jovanovich (undated edition).

Jung CG *et al. Man and His Symbols.* Garden City NY: Doubleday, 1964

Jung CG. *The Archetypes and the Collective Unconscious.* Collected Works 9(1); Princeton U. Press/ Bollingen, 1968

Jung CG. *Synchronicity: An Acausal Connecting Principle.*Princeton U. Press/ Bollingen, 1969; Collected Works 8:816-997

Kabat-Zinn J. *Full Catastrophe Living: Using the Wisdom of Your Body and Mind to Face Stress, Pain, and Illness.* New York: Delta/Dell, 1991.

Kabat-Zinn J. *Wherever You Go There You Are: Mindfulness Meditation in Everyday Life.* Hyperion, 1994.

Kabat-Zinn J *et al.* Four year follow-up of a meditation-based program for the self-regulation of chronic pain: Treatment outcomes and compliance. *Clinical Journal of Pain,* 1986; 2: 259-173.

Kahn D, Krippner S, Combs A. Dreaming and the self-organizing brain. *J. Consc. Studies,* 2000; 7: 4-11

Kaku M. *Hyperspace.* New York: Oxford University Press, 1994

Keating T. *Open Mind, Open Heart* (1986). New York: Continuum, 1991.

Kiecolt-Glasser JK *et al.* Psychological influences on surgical recovery: Perspectives from psychoneuroimmunology. *Am Psychol,* 1998 (Nov); 53: 1209-1218

Kiecolt-Glasser JK *et al.* Hypnosis as a modulator of cellular immune dysregulation during acute stress. *Journal of Consulting and Clinical Psychology,* 2001 (Aug); 69: 674-682

Kirschner M, Gerhard J, Mitchison T. Molecular "vitalism". *Cell,* 2000 (Jan 7); 100: 79-88.

Koenig HG *et al.* Religion, spirituality and medicine: A rebuttal to skeptics. *Int J Psychiatry Med,* 1999; 29(2): 123-31.

Koenig HG, McCullough ME, Larson DB. *Handbook of Religion and Health.* New York: Oxford University Press, 2001. (1200 references)

Krizek TI. Surgery: Is it an impairing profession? *Journal of the American College of Surgeons,* 2002 ; 194: 352-366

Krucoff MW, *et al.* Integrative noetic therapies as adjuncts to percutaneous intervention during unstable coronary syndromes: Monitoring and actualization of noetic training (MANTRA) feasibility pilot. *American Heart Journal,* 2001; 142: 760-767.

Lederman, L with Teresi D. *The God Particle: If the Universe is the Answer, What is the Question?* New York, Bantam Doubleday/Delta, 1994

Linde K *et al.* Are the clinical effects of homeopathy placebo effects? A meta-analysis of placebo-controlled trials. *Lancet,* 1997 (20 Sept); 350: 834-843

Lloyd S. *Programming the Universe: A Quantum Computer Scientist Takes on the Cosmos.* New York, Knopf, 2006.

Lykken JD. Disappearing dimensions. *Nature,* 2001 (12 July); 412: 130-131.

Makikallio TH *et al.* Heart rate dynamics before spontaneous onset of ventricular fibrillation in patients with healed myocardial infarcts. *American Journal of Cardiology,* 1999: 83: 880-884

Michels R and Marzuk PM. Progress in psychiatry (in two parts). *New Eng J Med* 1993; 329: (I) 552-560, (II) 628-638.

Miller GE *et al.* Psychosocial predictors of natural killer cell mobilization during marital conflict. *Health Psychology,* 1999 (May); 18: 262-271

Moore T. *Care of the Soul: A Guide for Cultivating Depth and Sacredness in Everyday Life,* HarperCollins, 1992. p. xi.

Murphy M and Donovan S. *The Physical and Psychological Effects of Meditation: A Review of Contemporary Research with Comprehensive Bibliography.* Institute of Noetic Sciences, 1997.

Nadeau R and Kafatos M. *The Non-local Universe: The New Physics of Matter and Mind.* New York: Oxford University Press, 1999.

Nunn C. Archetypes and memes: Their structure, relationships and behavior. *J. Consc Studies,* 1998 ; 5: 344-354.

Nunn C. Collapse of a quantum field may affect brain function. *J. Consc Studies,* 1994 ; 1: 127-139

O'Laoire S. An experimental study of effects of distant, intercessory prayer on self-esteem, anxiety, and depression. *Alternative Therapies in Health and Medicine,* 1997; 3: 38-53.

O'Regan B, Hirshberg C. *Spontaneous Remission: An Annotated Bibliography.* Petaluma CA: Institute of Noetic Sciences, 1993

Pargament KI *et al.* Religious struggle as a predictor of mortality among medically ill elderly patients. *Archives of Internal Medicine,* 2001 (Aug 13/27); 161: 181-1885

Peat FD. *Synchronicity: The Bridge Between Matter and Mind.* New York: Bantam, 1987.

Penrose R. *The Emperor's New Mind.* New York: Oxford University Press, 1989

Penrose R. *Shadows of the Mind: A Search for the Missing Science of Consciousness,* New York: Oxford University Press, 1994

Petrie KJ, Booth RJ, Pennebaker JW. The immunological effects of thought suppression. *J Pers Soc Psychol,* 1998 (Nov); 75: 1264-1272

Petty PG. Consciousness: A neurosurgical perspective. *J. Consc. Studies,* 1998 ; 5: 86-96

Pribham KH. *J Consc Studies,* 1999; 6(5):19-42

Prose NS. Paying attention. *JAMA,* 2000 (7 Jun); 283: 2763.

Roberts L, Ahmed I, Hall S. Intercessory prayer for the alleviation of ill health. *Cochrane Database of Systematic Reviews,* (2): CD000368, 2000. (Review, computer file, 4 references)

Rosa L *et al.* A close look at therapeutic touch. *J Amer Med Assoc* 1998 (1 Apr); 279: 1005-1010.

Roukes M. Plenty of room indeed. *Scientific American,* 2001 (Sep); 285(3): 48-57

Rowe MA *et al.* Experimental violation of a Bell's inequality with efficient detection. *Nature,* 2001 (Feb 15); 409: 791-794.

Schlitz M. Frontiers of research: Bridging worlds and filling gaps in the science of healing. Institute of Noetic Sciences: *Noetic Sciences Review,* 2002 (Mar-May); Number 59: 36-39.

Schlitz M and Braud W. Distant intentionality and healing: Assessing the evidence. *Alternative Therapies in Health and Medicine,* 1997; 3: 62-73. (65 references)

Schlosshauer M. Lifting the fog from the north. *Nature* 453, 39 (1 May 2008)

Schweitzer A. *The Words of Albert Schweitzer selected by Norman Cousins,* Newmarket Press, 1984.

Shear J. Experiential clarification of the problem of self. *Journal of Consciousness Studies,* 1998; 5: 673-686.

Sheldrake R. *A New Science of Life: The Hypothesis of Morphic Resonance* (1981). Rochester VT: Park Street Press, 1995.

Sheldrake R. *The Presence of The Past: Morphic Resonance and the Habits of Nature* (1988). Rochester VT: Park Street Press, 1995.

Sheldrake R. Morphic Resonance and the Collective Unconscious. *Psychological Perspectives:* Part I, 1987; 18:9-25. II, 1987; 18:320-331. III, 1988; 19:64-78.

Singletary SE. A working model for the time sequence of genetic changes in breast tumorigenesis. *Journal of the American College of Surgeons,* 2002 (Feb); 194: 202-216.

Skelly, FJ. Decline and fall, an interview with Dr. Edward Shorter; *American Medical News,* Aug 3, 1992.

Sloan EP, Bagiella E, Powell T. Religion, spirituality and medicine. *Lancet,* 1999 (Feb 20): 353: 664-67.

Sloan EP. (Reply to correspondence.) *New Engl J Med,* 2000 (Nov 2); 343: 1341-42.

Sloan EP, *et al.* Should physicians prescribe religious activities? *New Engl J Med,* 2000 (Jun 22): 342: 1913-16.

Smolin L. *The Life of the Cosmos.* New York: Oxford University Press, 1997

Smolin L. *Three Roads to Quantum Gravity.* New York: Basic Books, 2001

Spiegel D. Embodying the mind in psychooncology research. *Advances in Mind-Body Medicine,* 1999; 15: 267-273.

Spiegel D *et al.* Effect of psychosocial treatment on survival of patients with metastatic breast cancer. *Lancet,* 1989; 2(8668): 888-891

Squires E. Quantum theory and the need for consciousness. *J. Consc. Studies,* 1994; 1: 201-204.

Stapp HP. On quantum theories of the mind. *J Consc Studies,* 1999; 6: 61-65

Stevens A. *Archetypes: A Natural History of the Self.* New York: Quill, 1983

Targ E. Evaluating distant healing: A research review. *Alternative Therapies in Health and Medicine,* 1997; 3: 74-78.

Taylor WR. A 'periodic table' for protein structures. *Nature,* 2002 (11 April); 416: 657-660

Teilhard de Chardin, P. *The Phenomenon of Man.* New York: Harper/Colophon, 1975

Veltman, MJG. The Higgs Boson. *Scientific American* 1986 (Nov); 76-84

Vikman S *et al.* Differences in heart rate dynamics before the spontaneous onset of long and short episodes of paroxysmal atrial fibrillation. *Annals of Noninvasive Electrocardiology,* 2001; 6: 134-142

Waldfogel S. Spirituality in medicine. *Primary Care,* 1997; 24: 963-976.

Walker SR *et al.* Intercessory prayer in the treatment of alcohol abuse and dependence: a pilot investigation. *Alternative Therapies in Health and Medicine,* 1997; 3: 79-86

Wang ZS *et al.* Spatio-temporal nonlinear modeling of gastric myoelectrical activity. *Methods of Information in Medicine,* 2000 (Jun); 39: 186-190

Whitehead AN. *Process and Reality.* New York: Macmillan, 1929

Whitfield J. All creatures great and small. *Nature,* 2001 (27 Sep); 413: 342-344

Wickramasekera I. Secrets kept from the mind but not the body or behavior: the unsolved problems of identifying and treating somatization and psychophysiological disease. *Advances in Mind-Body Medicine,* 1998; 14:81-98.

Wilber K. *Sex, Ecology, Spirituality: The Spirit of Evolution.* Boston: Shambhala, 1995.

Wiseman R and Schlitz M. Experimenter effects and the remote detection of staring. *Journal of Parapsychology,* 1997; 61: 197-208.

Wolfram S. *A New Kind of Science.* Wolfram Media, 2002.

Yeragani VK *et al.* Nonlinear measures of heart period variability: Decreased measures of symbolic dynamics in patients with panic disorder. *Depression & Anxiety,* 2000; 12: 67-77

Zewail AH. The fog that was not. *Nature,* 2001 (19 July); 412: 279.

Zurek WH. Sub-Planck structure in phase space and its relevance for quantum decoherence. *Nature,* 2001 (16 Aug); 412: 712-717

Zurek WH. Decoherence and the transition from quantum to classical. *Physics Today,* 1991;44(10): 36-44

about the author

Dr. Bessinger, now retired, practiced surgery in South Carolina. He has written medical journal articles and editorials about philosophy, medical ethics, international health programs, and clinical practice, and books—poetry, ethics, and religion and science. He has won the Roe Foundation Award for medical writing. His global perspective and interest in integrative studies are shaped, in large part, by diverse medical experiences in New England, Hawaii, the Philippines, Antarctica, and Haiti.

current website

dbScriptorium
http://home.earthlink.net/~dbscr/

www.ingramcontent.com/pod-product-compliance
Lightning Source LLC
Chambersburg PA
CBHW051545170526
45165CB00002B/894